NAILS, **NAILS**, NAILS!

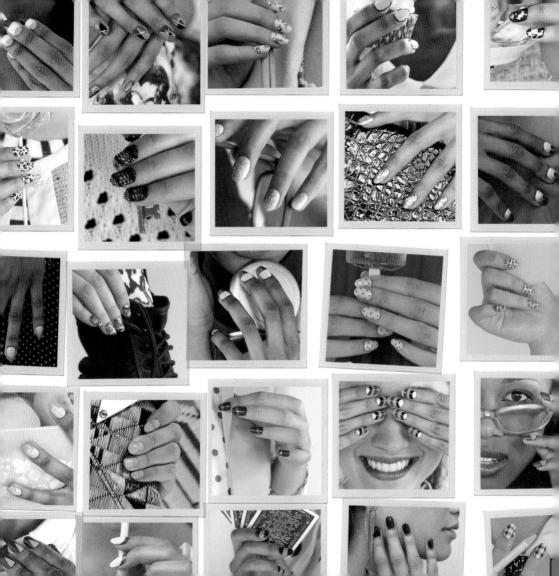

NAILS, **NAILS,** NAILS!

25 CREATIVE DIY NAIL ART PROJECTS

Madeline Poole

PHOTOGRAPHS BY LARA ROSSIGNOL

CHRONICLE BOOKS

SAN FRANCISCO

Library of Congress Cataloging-in-Publication Data available.

ISBN: 978-1-4521-1902-1

Manufactured in China

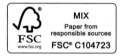

Design by Alicia Pompei
Wardrobe styling by Shiffy Kagan
Wardrobe and props from Nasty Gal, Traveler's Bookcase,
    Polkadots & Moonbeams, and Marie Turnor Accessories
Makeup and hair styling by Wendy Osmundson
Models from M Model Management
This book has been set in Avant Garde Gothic, Miller, and Prestige.

10 9 8 7

Chronicle Books LLC
680 Second Street
San Francisco, California 94107
www.chroniclebooks.com

To my family—

Nancy, Tom, Hannah,
Jaime, Lucy, Sally, Joey,
Aya, and Lola

Contents

Introduction

I'm often asked why nail art is so popular these days—why people of all ages, backgrounds, and fashion sensibilities are experimenting with unexpected colors and bold, eye-catching designs. There are as many different answers to this question as there are ways of painting your nails. Too many to count! But one thing is clear—nail art is fun. *Really* fun. It's as simple as that.

Nail art is where art, beauty, and fashion unite. Many people come to nail art with an interest in cosmetics, applying polish and colors with the same passion and precision as they do eyeliner and lipstick. Others view it as a fashion accessory, completing an outfit and balancing color and texture in the same way a hat or purse can be a stylish finishing touch. Still others enjoy it as an exciting craft, spontaneously arranging shapes and colors on the nail like paints on a canvas, patches on a quilt, or beads on a necklace.

For me, nail art is a form of self-expression that channels all my hobbies and interests: miniature painting, color theory, pattern, and of course fashion and beauty. My nail art toolbox includes a wide range of inspirations: ancient symbols, optical illusions, textiles, pop art, nature, iconography, murals, sculpture, and music, among many others. When it comes to self-expression, anything goes! Inspiration can be found in the most unexpected places.

As you complete the projects in this book, I hope you will find new ways of expressing yourself and new ways of using nail polish that you never imagined. Start by reading the tools and techniques sections for helpful nail art know-how. Then choose from the twenty-five classic and original designs that represent a broad range of styles. Many projects require only nail polish, while some feature embellishments such as crystals, lace, and even shimmering gold leaf. Some play tricks on the eye—like Brick (page 91) and Electric Fade (page 111)—while others are stunningly simple, like Pyramid Point (page 103), 1920s Two-Tone (page 43), and Half-Moon (page 27). Find a partner to complete the more challenging styles—Plaid (page 123), Cubic (page 71), and Multistripe (page 119), for example—as extra hands are needed to apply intricate details. All projects offer opportunity for your own customization and interpretation.

Let each project be an experiment. If you make a mistake, simply wipe it off and start over—or keep going, and see where it takes you. Let each nail you decorate represent a different side of your personality. Your finished nails will be stylish, crafty, beautiful, and uniquely yours, all at once.

—*Madeline Poole*

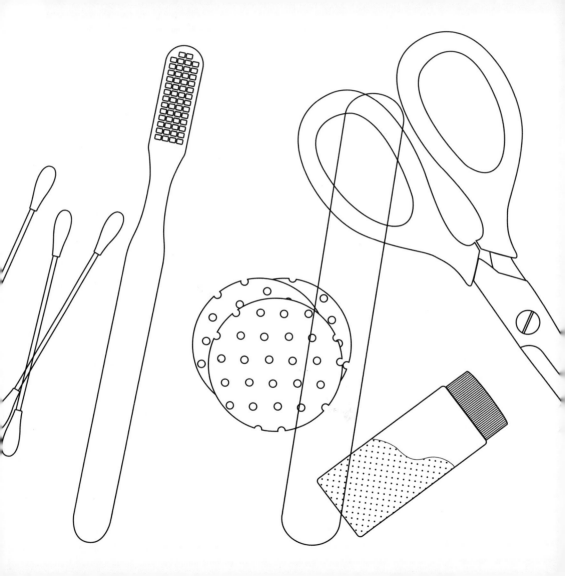

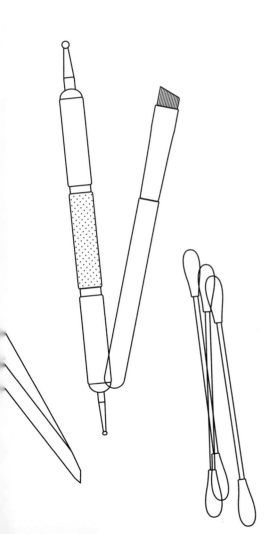

**BEFORE
YOU
BEGIN . . .**

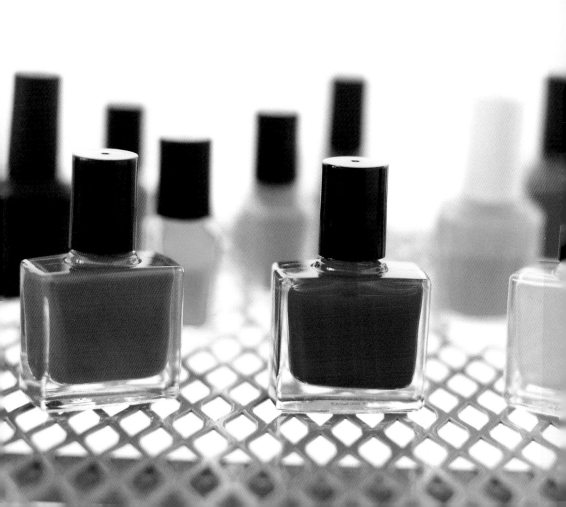

Nail Art Tools

There are dozens of nail art tools on the market, many of which are common household items or craft supplies that you might already own. The following lists include the key tools that every aspiring nail artist should obtain, plus miscellaneous items that are used in the projects in this book.

POLISHES

Clear base coat creates a smooth first layer before color is applied and aids in polish bonding to the nail.

Clear top coat is a glossy sealant that provides a protective layer for the completed look and adds gorgeous shine. A fast-drying top coat is a must.

Nail polish or nail varnish is a lacquer that applies color to the nail.

A **striper polish** is a nail polish featuring a brush that is long and thin, perfect for painting stripes (as its name implies), intricate curves, and covering larger areas of miniature decoration. Stripers are available in a wide variety of colors, just like nail polishes.

BASIC TOOLS

An **angled-edge eyeliner brush**, typically used on the eyes, is recommended as a nail art tool for applying nail polish remover with precision. (It is important to designate one brush for the exclusive purpose of nail art. For safety and sanitary reasons, do not use one brush on both nails and eyes.)

A **cotton swab**, with the tip thickly coated with nail polish, can be used like a stamp to create organic round shapes on the nail.

A **disposable white plastic plate** makes an excellent painter's palette, providing a clean, flat surface for polish puddles.

A **double-sided dotting tool** features round metal knobs at each end. Dip them in polish and apply to the nail to create small dots and perfect circles. The knobs can also be used to apply individual pieces of glitter and crystals to the nail.

A **nail file** is used to shape natural nails before polish is applied.

Nail glue adheres crystals and other embellishments to the nail.

Nail polish remover is key! Do not attempt a nail art project without it. Apply polish remover before, during, and after projects as needed.

Paper reinforcements are an office supply item used in nail art to create a smooth outline of the moon area. The standard size (with a center hole that is ¼ in/6 mm in diameter) is most suitable for these projects.

A **plastic soda cap** is handy for holding small amounts of nail polish remover, providing convenient, instant access to this crucial cleanup tool.

Keep **scissors** on hand for when cutting is needed—while preparing clear sticky tape for stenciling, for example, or cutting lace and other nail decorations.

Sticky tape—such as clear packaging tape and masking tape—can be used like a stencil. Cut it into strips and shapes and apply it to the natural, unpolished nail. When painted over, they help create smooth lines and clean shapes. (Do not apply tape to a wet nail, as the tape can damage underlying polish.)

A **toothbrush** can be used as a coarse paintbrush, to splatter polish on the nail, creating marbled or sprayed effects on the nail. (For obvious health and safety reasons, it is important to designate one brush for the exclusive purpose of nail art.)

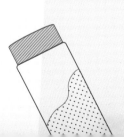
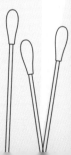

Toothpicks can be used for painting tiny dots, and for applying individual pieces of glitter to the nail if a dotting tool is not available.

Tweezers have multiple uses in nail art, primarily acting as an extension of your fingers as you allow wet nails to dry. Use them to pick up tiny decorative crystals and transfer them to the nail, or to remove adhesive strips from the nail with precision.

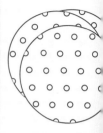

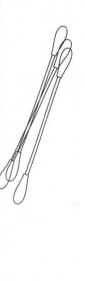

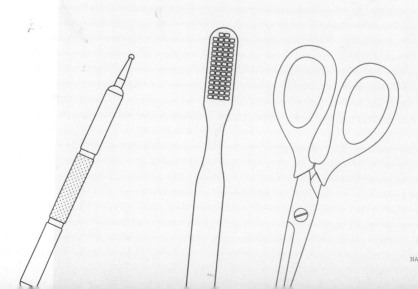

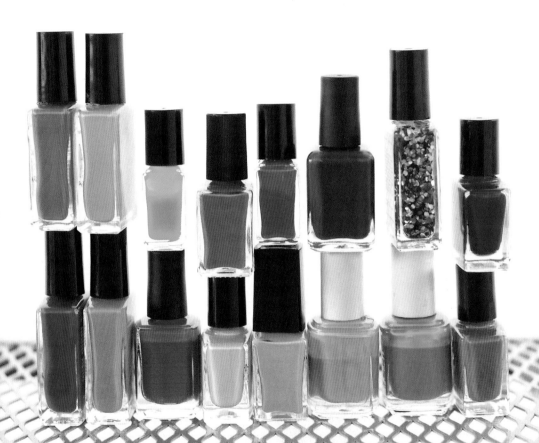

Nail Art Techniques

POLISHES

Nail polish is the true hero of any nail art look. Nothing has quite the pop, sheen, or luxurious finish of colorful, polished nails. The vast selection of polish colors on the market lets you customize your look to suit any mood or outfit. Build and maintain your collection using the following tips, and as you browse the projects in this book, note that you can substitute your own color selections. Remember, anything goes!

Choosing Polishes

Opaque polishes work best for nail art because they require fewer coats than translucent polishes. The best way to test the opacity of a polish is to try it out, painting a single stroke down the center of one of your nails. Can you see the nail through the polish, or does the polish cover the nail in a dense layer of color? If you are shopping for polishes where testers are not available, simply hold the bottle up to ceiling light and tilt it sideways. If light easily passes through the glass, then the polish has low opacity.

A quality associated with opaqueness is pigmentation, meaning the concentration of individual units of color. Polishes with high opacity are likely to have high pigment count. As you grow your nail polish collection, choose several polishes that are highly opaque and highly pigmented.

Keep in mind that opacity and pigmentation have little to do with color darkness and lightness. Light-colored polishes, such as white and pale pink, can be just as opaque and highly pigmented as dark polishes, and vice versa. Likewise, the thickness of a polish is not an indicator of opacity. In fact, thick, syrupy polishes are most likely old and should just be tossed out!

Storing Polishes

Nail polishes expire after a year or two. Exposure to changing temperatures and humidity can alter the consistency of a polish, so storing in a bathroom is not recommended. Make a safe home for your nail art supplies in a closet and store the bottles upright and securely capped.

Applying Base and Top Coats

A clear base coat (also called a primer) is applied to clean, unpainted nails before colored polish is added. The primer creates a smooth clear layer on which to begin painting and provides greater adhesion for the polish. It is commonly applied during nail art but is not a necessity. A clear top coat, however, is vital—it's the perfect finishing touch to any nail art project. Applied at the very end, it seals the underlying polish and provides protection, durability, and a glossy shine. Be sure to use a fast-drying clear top coat, which reduces the final drying time of the completed look.

CREATING YOUR WORKSPACE

The most important thing to consider as you choose a workspace is keeping the surrounding area clean and protecting furniture and surfaces from polish spills and stains. Choose a table or other sturdy flat surface and cover with white waxed paper, taping down the edges of the paper to keep it secure. Make sure your waxed paper surface is large enough to contain two spread hands plus all your nail art supplies, with some extra space. Arrange your nail preparation supplies—such as nail files, clippers, and nail polish remover—to your front left, and nail art supplies—such as polishes and brushes—to your front right. (Reverse if left-handed.) Keep a small stack of paper towels and a small trash can nearby.

Your workspace should be well-lit and well-ventilated. Open a window or use a small fan to disperse polish and polish remover odors. When not in use, store nail art supplies in small plastic bins or shoeboxes, all in one place for easy access.

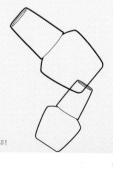

NAIL PREPARATION

Nail preparation can be extensive, including a full range of manicure procedures, or it can be as simple as you like. The projects in this book require merely a thorough cleaning of the hands. First, remove old nail polish with nail polish remover and a clean cotton pad. Then wash hands with soap and water. If you would like to clip or file your nails, do so now, and follow with a second hand-washing using soap and water. Dry hands thoroughly with a cloth towel. Apply a clear base coat, allow it to dry, and you're ready to begin!

DRYING TIME

As mentioned previously, a fast-drying clear top coat is a must for any nail art project. A single coat is all that is needed. All projects in this book include a top coat as the final step, along with a 15-minute period of stillness when hands should be laid flat and undisturbed. (Do not shake hands to speed up the drying time, as this can unsettle the polish.) After 15 minutes, touch nails lightly to confirm they are dry. Hands can then be used for light tasks, but wait an extra 25 minutes before increasing activity, not letting your nails come in direct contact with objects that could dent or smudge the nail art.

For most nail art projects, multiple coats and multiple colors are applied to each nail, and underlying layers should be dry before the next coat or color is applied. However, drying time between coats is much shorter than drying time of a completed look. If nails are dry to a light touch, generally after a few minutes, they are ready for the next layer of polish.

KEEPING CLEAN AND CLEANUP

Your Workspace

A messy workspace can create mess-ups on the nail and a mess all over your hands. An organized workspace, with all the supplies you need right there at your fingertips, is key to keeping clean. Prevent a mess from accumulating by tidying up as you go—closing polish bottles after you apply color and discarding used paper products, for example—but save the major cleanup until your nails are completely dry.

Your Nails

Easy access to nail polish remover is a must for nail art projects. Before beginning a project, apply it to the nail area using a clean cotton pad to remove old polish and natural skin oils. Apply it during a project if a mess arises. And apply it after completing a project to remove stray polish from the cuticle area. A small angled-edge eyeliner brush allows you to apply remover with precision, and the brush handle keeps a protective distance between your working hand and the powerful remover.

Before you start a project, pour some polish remover into a plastic soda cap, and place it next to the angled-edge eyeliner brush. As needed, simply dip the brush into the polish remover, press lightly against a paper towel to soak up excess, and apply to the areas of the cuticle where you see stray polish. However, avoid overusing your hands during projects, as you will likely have wet polish on your nails that needs time to set and dry. Instead, save minor nail cleanup for the end, after all nail art has been applied. Just before adding the top coat, do a quick review of fingers and cuticle area, and carefully wipe away messes with the angled-edge brush, dipping into the remover as needed.

OPTIONS AND ALTERNATIVES

Like any craft or beauty regime, nail art has its secrets. The tips that follow will broaden your skills, amp up the fun factor, and extend the life of your finished, gorgeous nails—and make your friends ask, "How did you do that?"

Embellishments

An exciting aspect of nail art is the use of embellishments—decorative materials that can be adhered to the nail to add unexpected texture, dimension, and novelty. Some projects in this book feature embellishments for brilliant, sparkling effect, such as Glitter Studs (page 67) and Half Nail with Crystals (page 95). In the Gold Leaf project (page 31), small pieces of shimmering metal foil are nestled in black polish, while the Lace project (page 107) calls for real pieces of lace. There are few limits to what you can apply to the nail, using clear top coat or nail glue as an adhesive. Think sequins, feathers, torn bits of colored paper, seed beads, stickers, and even flower petals.

False Nails

Many nail art looks, including some of the projects in this book, take a long time to produce and require intricate handiwork.

If you want to preserve the nail art and reuse it—rather than wiping it all away with polish remover when it's time for a change—then simply apply nail art to a set of false nails and enjoy them again and again.

Another benefit of false nails is that both hands are free to complete the look. (Decorate the false nails before attaching them to your real nails for the cleanest result.) If your nails are naturally short, false nails will give you more length to work with, much like a painter deciding to use a larger canvas. False nails can even be filed and shaped just like natural nails. All the projects in this book can be applied to false nails, which you can store in small ziplock bags. Choose a set of false nails that are a natural, unpainted color and read instructions carefully before proceeding to nail art projects.

PARTNER PROJECTS

- -

Many projects in this book are recommended for two people, for greater precision and cleaner shapes—and for the fun of it! For example, Flame (page 79) and Outline (page 55) involve more challenging techniques and feature intricate details that would be quite difficult to apply to your own nails using just one hand. For partner projects, sit across from your partner while you apply designs to their nails, and then let them return the favor.

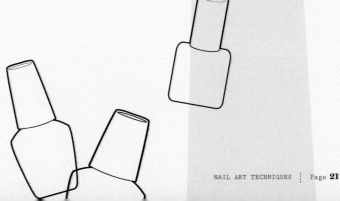

Nail Anatomy

THE SIX BASIC AREAS OF THE NAIL ARE:

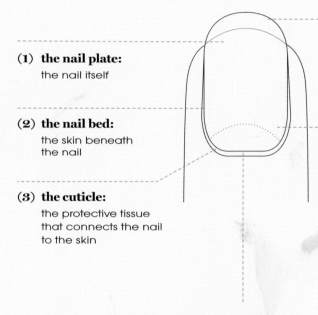

(1) the nail plate:
the nail itself

(2) the nail bed:
the skin beneath
the nail

(3) the cuticle:
the protective tissue
that connects the nail
to the skin

(4) the tip:
the part of the nail that
extends beyond the skin

**(5) the lunula,
or the "moon":**
the pale, crescent-
shaped area peeking
out from the bottom
of the nail. For most
people, the moon is
most visible on the
thumb and often not
visible at all on other
fingers.

(6) the edge: where the nail meets the cuticle

Quick Tips:

Before you begin a nail art project, here are a few quick tips and reminders for a fabulous finished look every time:

- *Review the previous sections—Nail Art Tools, Nail Art Techniques, and Nail Anatomy—for expert results and to avoid interruptions and oversights during the projects.*

- *Use nail polishes that are new and fresh, with a smooth liquid consistency.*

- *Unless otherwise specified, these projects make use of the brush that comes in the nail polish bottle.*

- *For precision and cleanliness, use as few strokes as possible when applying color.*

- *For looks that make use of multiple layers of polish colors, always apply colors with thinner coverage first.*

- *If you have applied the suggested number of polish coats and the color coverage is not opaque enough, apply another coat.*

HALF-MOON

GOLD LEAF

CHAIN LINK

NEGATIVE SPACE

1920S TWO-TONE

LEOPARD

CLASSIC CAMO

OUTLINE

MOSAIC

NAUTICAL

GLITTER STUDS

CUBIC

ABSTRACT FLORAL

FLAME

TRIPLE ECLIPSE

SPRAY PAINT

BRICK

HALF NAIL
WITH CRYSTALS

STUDDED
ECLIPSE

PYRAMID
POINT

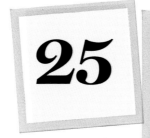

25

**DIY
NAIL ART
PROJECTS**

LACE

ELECTRIC FADE

JEWEL-ENCRUSTED

MULTISTRIPE

PLAID

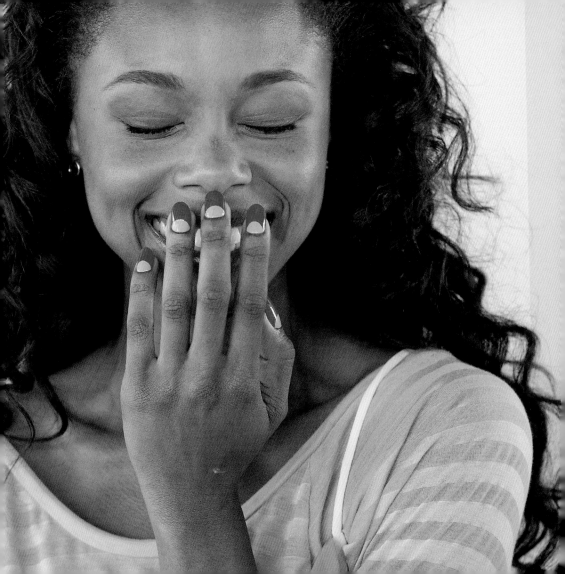

Half-Moon

This is a girly yet grown-up look, featuring painted crescents and retro color contrast. Color-coordinate it with your outfit for two-toned fun.

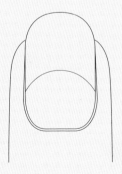

Tools:

- ☐ Pink polish
- ☐ Clear top coat
- ☐ Paper reinforcements
- ☐ Red polish
- ☐ Tweezers

(continued)

Half-Moon Instructions

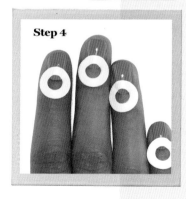

Note:

This look can feature any color pairing, but make sure the top color polish is opaque enough to cover the bottom color.

Step 1

Apply one coat of pink polish to all nails and allow to dry.

Step 2

Apply a second coat of pink polish to the bottom of each nail, carefully covering the moon area (see Nail Anatomy, page 22) and painting to the edges of the bottom part of the nail. Allow time to dry.

Step 3

Apply a clear top coat to all nails and allow 20 minutes to dry.

Step 4

Position a paper reinforcement on the bottom of each nail so the top of the reinforcement follows the line of the moon area and covers the bottom one-third of the nail. Press lightly so the paper reinforcement adheres to the nail, pressing more firmly at the edges of the nail where it meets the cuticle.

Step 5

Paint the nail with red polish using upward strokes, swiping your brush across the top of the paper reinforcement and continuing to the top of the nail. Apply to all nails and allow to dry, then repeat with a second coat of red polish.

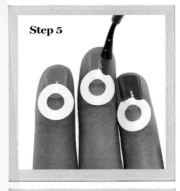

Step 6

When polish is completely dry, use tweezers to remove the paper reinforcements, pulling slowly and carefully from one side to the other.

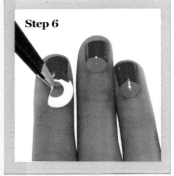

Step 7

Apply clear top coat and allow the completed look to dry.

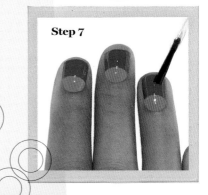

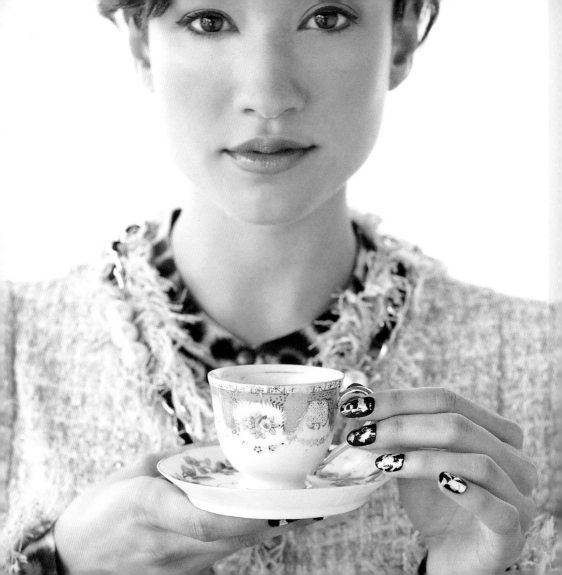

Gold Leaf

Glimmering gold leaf shines against velvety black for dramatic, old-world elegance. This look is all about special occasions, from the red carpet to a candlelit dinner.

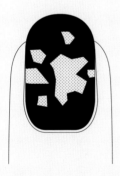

Tools:

- ☐ Gold leaf flakes
- ☐ Tweezers (optional)
- ☐ Black polish
- ☐ Angled-edge eyeliner brush (completely dry)
- ☐ Clear top coat

(continued)

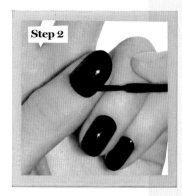

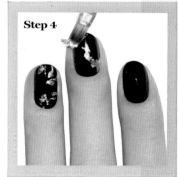

Gold Leaf Instructions

Step 1

Pour gold leaf flakes onto your workspace and space them out so you can clearly see the size and shape of each individual piece. Pieces smaller than ¼ in/6 mm wide will work best for this project. (Use tweezers or your fingernails to tear larger pieces into smaller sizes.)

Step 2

Apply one coat of black polish to all nails and allow to dry.

Step 3

Apply a second coat of black polish to one nail and allow it to dry for 60 seconds. The slightly wet polish will act as an adhesive for the gold leaf.

Step 4

Use the angled-edge eyeliner brush to pick up a large piece of gold leaf by lightly touching it with the bristles. Transfer it to the wet nail, placing it wherever you like and gently pressing down with the bristles until the gold leaf adheres. Do not let the bristles touch the wet polish, and don't worry if the gold leaf is crinkly—that is its natural appearance.

Step 5

Repeat step 4, applying a medium-size piece of gold leaf to the nail, followed by a smaller piece. Allow to dry.

Step 6

Proceed to the next nail, repeating steps 3 to 5 until all nails feature gold leaf.

Step 7

When dry, apply clear top coat and allow the completed look to dry.

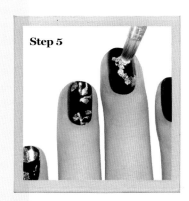

Step 5

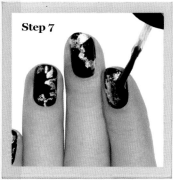

Step 7

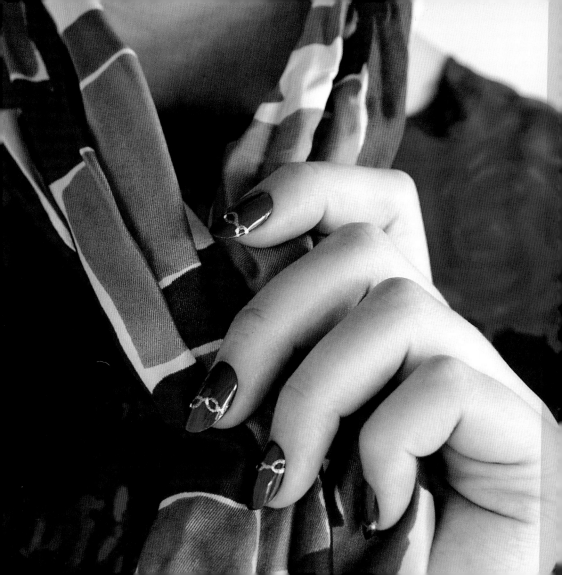

Chain Link

Fingertips are draped in gold in this grown-up, opulent style. Raid your grandmother's closet for bright silk scarves or pair with a blazer for a truly high-polish look.

Partner recommended.

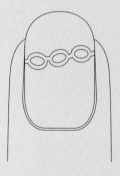

Tools:

- ☐ Royal blue polish
- ☐ Gold striper polish
- ☐ White striper polish
- ☐ Clear top coat

(continued)

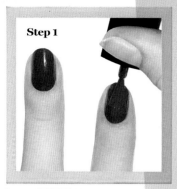

Step 1

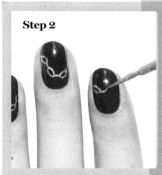

Step 2

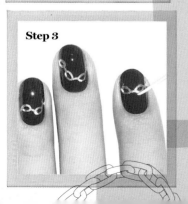

Step 3

Chain Link Instructions

Note:
Customize this look by creating chains of different sizes or painting larger or smaller connected shapes. Find a favorite gold necklace and use it as inspiration.

Step 1

Apply two coats of royal blue polish to all nails and allow to dry after each coat.

Step 2

With the gold striper polish, create chain links by painting connected circles or ovals across the nail. Proceed to the next nail, changing the direction or curve of the chain. Apply to all nails and allow to dry.

Step 3

With the white striper polish, add a white accent to the corner of each chain link by lightly touching the white tip to the nail. Apply to the same corner of each link to give the impression of light reflecting off the chain. Apply to all nails and allow to dry.

Step 4

Apply clear top coat and allow the completed look to dry.

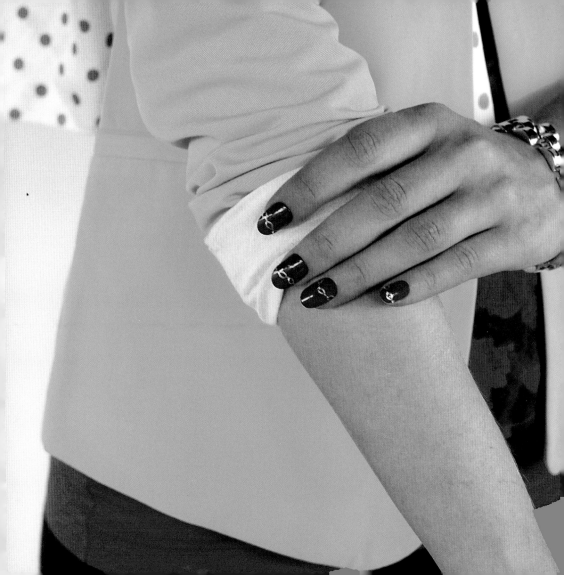

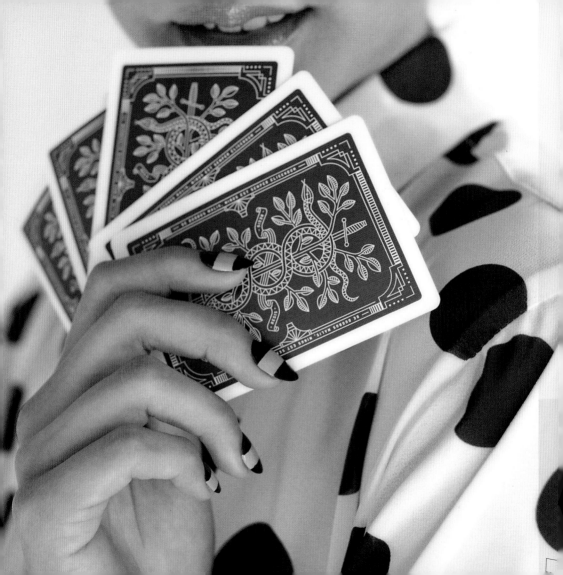

Negative Space

The natural nail is the star of this edgy, futuristic style. Use black polish for subtle self-expression or bright, bold polishes for a color-blocking effect.

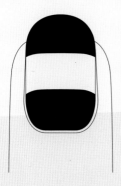

Tools:

☐ Scissors

☐ Sticky tape (preferably masking tape)

☐ Tweezers

☐ Black polish

☐ Angled-edge eyeliner brush (optional)

☐ Nail polish remover (optional)

☐ Paper towel (optional)

☐ Clear top coat

(continued)

Negative Space Instructions

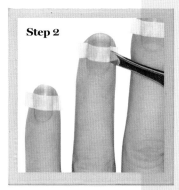
Step 2

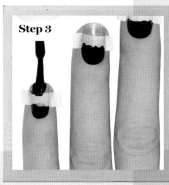
Step 3

Note:

Customize this look by changing the size of the pieces of tape, which will reduce or enlarge the amount of negative space on the nail.

Step 1

With scissors, cut ten pieces of masking tape. Each piece should be slightly longer than the width of your nail, and ⅛ in/4 mm wide. Lightly stick pieces to the edge of a table surface until needed.

Step 2

With tweezers, pick up one piece of tape at a time and place a strip horizontally across the middle of each unpainted nail. Press firmly, and use tweezers to press tape into the edges where the nail meets the cuticles.

Step 3

Apply black polish to all nails, painting the bottom half and then the top half, using upward strokes. Take care along the edges of the tape so polish does not leak under the tape. Allow to dry, then apply a second coat.

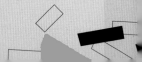

Step 4

When polish is completely dry, use tweezers to remove the strips of tape, pulling slowly and carefully from one side to another.

Step 5

If polish has leaked under the tape, leaving behind a jagged line, dip the angled-edge eyeliner brush into polish remover, press against a paper towel to soak up excess, and apply the bristles to the area for precise cleanup.

Step 6

Apply clear top coat and allow the completed look to dry.

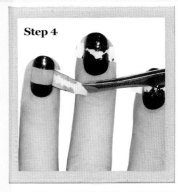

Step 4

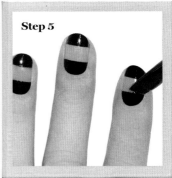

Step 5

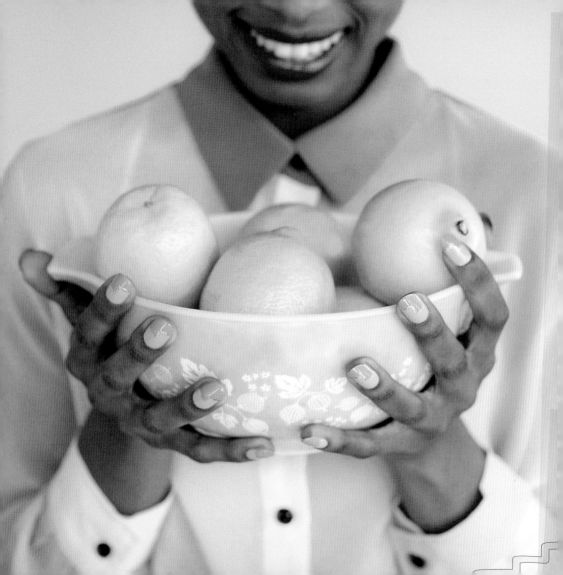

1920s Two-Tone

This project is all about looking gorgeous and having a good time—Gatsby-style. Celebrate your inner flapper with sleek, glittery angles. Wear with sequins and loose, short dresses, or pair it with a casual outfit for the perfect touch of vintage glam.

Partner recommended.

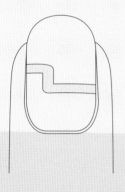

Tools:

- ☐ Aqua polish
- ☐ Ochre or bright yellow polish
- ☐ Gold glitter striper polish
- ☐ Clear top coat

(continued)

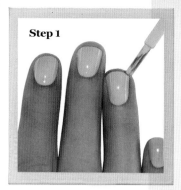

Step 1

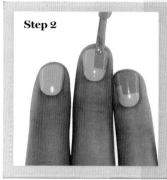

Step 2

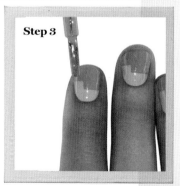

Step 3

1920s Two-Tone Instructions

Step 1

Apply two coats of aqua polish to all nails and allow to dry after each coat.

Step 2

With the ochre polish, paint a rectangle in the top right corner of the nail, starting at the right cuticle, just below the midline of the nail, and continuing up to the tip of the nail. Then paint a shorter rectangle in the top left corner, starting halfway up the side of the neighboring rectangle and continuing up to the tip of the nail. Complete all ten nails and allow to dry.

Step 3

Repeat step 2, applying a second coat of ochre polish to all nails, and allow to dry.

Step 4

With the gold glitter striper polish, paint carefully over the zigzag line where the two colors of polish meet. Apply to all nails and allow to dry. Repeat this step until you have achieved the glitter density that you like.

Step 5

When dry, apply clear top coat and allow the completed look to dry.

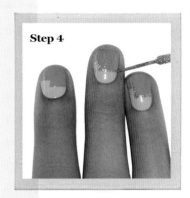

Step 4

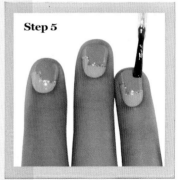

Step 5

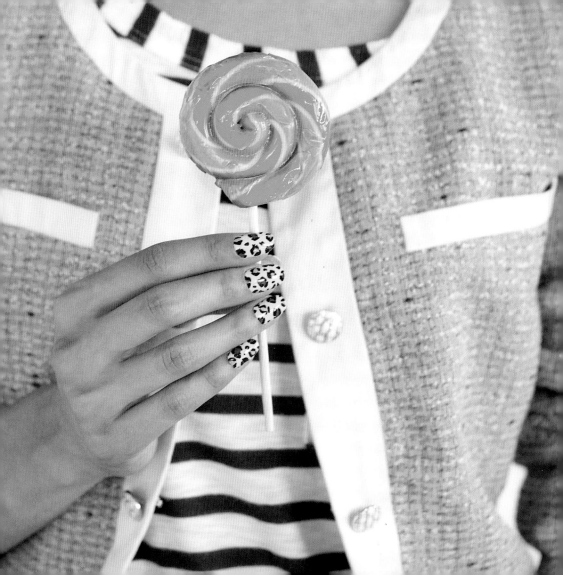

Leopard

Pop art goes on safari in this updated classic look, featuring traditional spots and unexpected primary colors. Fun to make and always stylish, there's nothing that doesn't pair well with leopard. Lollipops, anyone?

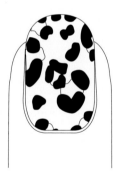

Tools:

- ☐ Yellow polish
- ☐ Red striper polish
- ☐ Blue striper polish
- ☐ Black striper polish
- ☐ Clear top coat

(continued)

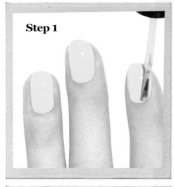

Leopard Instructions

Step 1

Apply two coats of yellow polish to all nails and allow to dry after each coat.

Step 2

With the red striper polish, paint two or three spots of red on each nail. Spots can be any shape—circles, ovals, curves, splotches—and they don't need to have a precise edge. Apply to all nails and allow to dry.

Step 3

Repeat step 2 with blue striper polish, leaving empty yellow space in between dots.

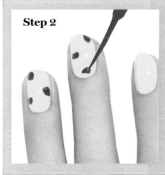

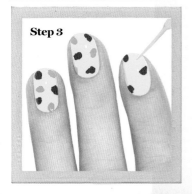

Step 4

With the black striper polish, paint two or three curved, uneven lines around the edge of each spot but do not encircle the spots completely. Then, if you like, you can paint small black dots and squiggles in areas that are empty of decoration. Apply to all nails.

Step 5

When dry, apply clear top coat and allow the completed look to dry.

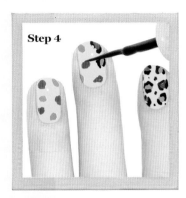

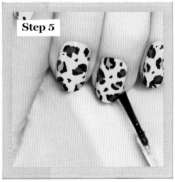

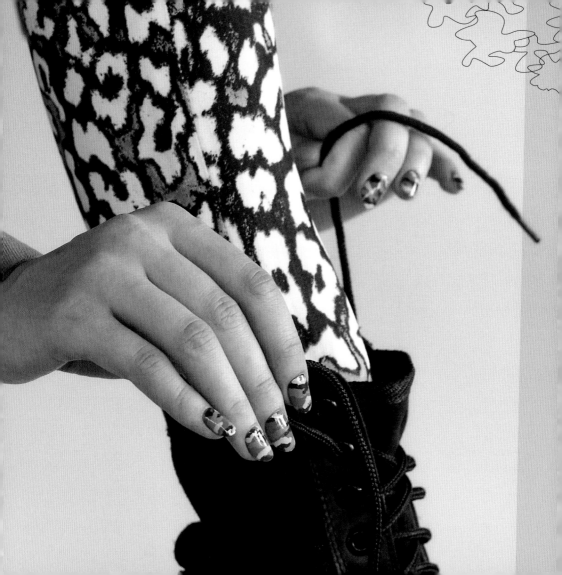

Classic Camo

Here's a great everyday look for tackling your to-do list, fighting crowds at the mall, or catching an action movie with friends. Feminize with metal jewelry and layered gold chains, or take the stealth approach with cargos and comfy flats.

Partner recommended.

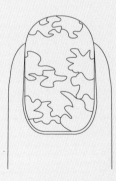

Tools:

☐ Three shades of green polish (kelly green, army green, and dark green)

☐ Beige polish

☐ Clear top coat

(continued)

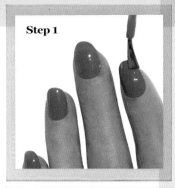

Step 1

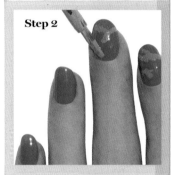

Step 2

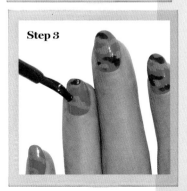

Step 3

Classic Camo Instructions

Step 1

Apply two coats of kelly green polish to all nails and allow to dry after each coat.

Step 2

Using the army green polish, apply one squiggly line to each nail, creating a shape like a tree trunk with two or three branches. Create different-looking tree shapes on each nail by changing their direction—some growing vertically, for example, while others run diagonally across the nail. Do not let tree shapes go all the way from end to end of the nail. Rather, paint branches in errant directions, leaving plenty of space around each branch. Allow nails to dry.

Step 3

Apply random patches of dark green polish along the edges of the army green branches. Apply to all nails and allow to dry.

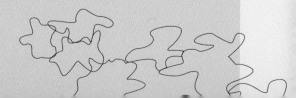

Step 4

Repeat step 3 using beige polish.

Step 5

When dry, apply clear top coat and allow the completed look to dry.

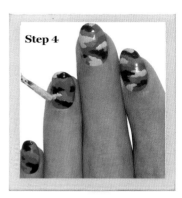

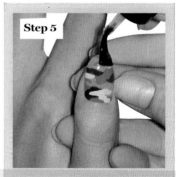

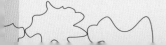

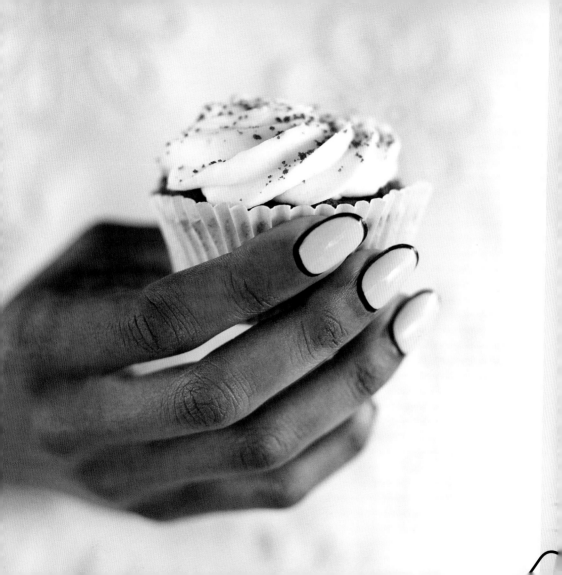

Outline

Yummy up your nails with sweet, layered ovals, stacked and frosted smooth like a cake. This look is perfect for a party!

Partner recommended.

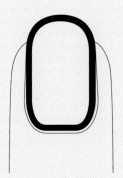

Tools:

- ☐ Black striper polish
- ☐ Pink polish
- ☐ Clear top coat

    (continued)

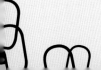

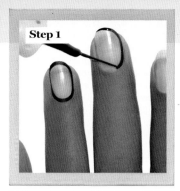

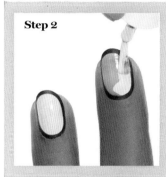

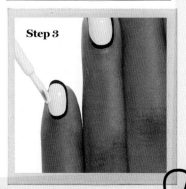

Outline Instructions

Step 1

With the black striper polish, paint a fine line around the edge of the entire nail, creating an oval outline. Apply to all nails and allow to dry, and apply a second coat if stronger coverage is needed. (Don't worry if your outline is slightly uneven—you will perfect the shape in the steps that follow.)

Step 2

Fill in the interior ovals with pink polish. First, carefully create a pink outline immediately inside the black outline, using circular strokes: start by painting a curve from the bottom of the outline to the top, then along the tip of the nail from left to right, and then from top to bottom. Fill in the center of the pink outline with pink polish, again using circular strokes. Apply to all nails and allow to dry.

Step 3

Apply another coat of pink to all nails, polishing inside the black outline, and allow to dry.

Step 4

Before applying clear top coat, review the black outline. If any part of it has lost its shape due to stray pink polish, carefully doctor it up with the black striper polish and allow to dry.

Step 5

Apply clear top coat and allow the completed look to dry.

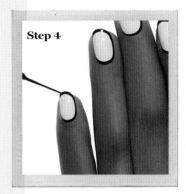

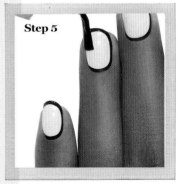

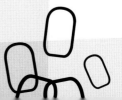

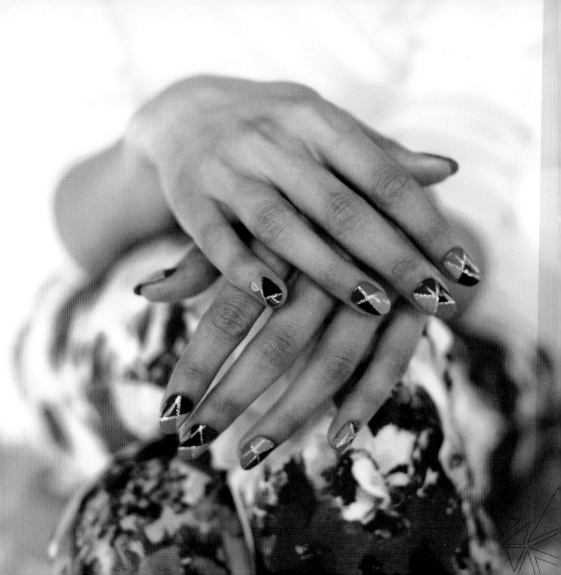

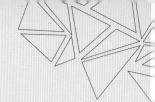

Mosaic

This look is cute and clever, with geometric patterns, sharp edges, and plenty of ways to customize. Make every nail look different by alternating shapes, then outline in gold for a kaleidoscopic effect.

Partner recommended.

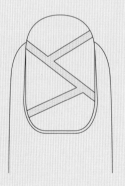

Tools:

☐ Red polish

☐ Maroon polish

☐ Pink polish

☐ Blue polish

☐ Gold glitter
striper polish

☐ Clear top coat

(continued)

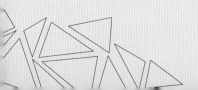

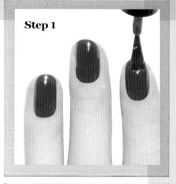

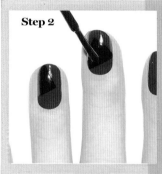

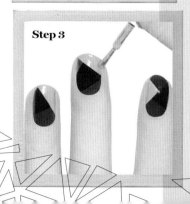

Mosaic Instructions

Note:

This look can feature any color assortment, but top color polishes should be opaque enough to cover the bottom color polishes.

Step 1

Apply one coat of red polish to all nails and allow to dry.

Step 2

Apply maroon polish to the nail in angular shapes. For example, paint one corner of the nail maroon, or add a maroon triangle to one side of the nail. Make every nail look different by getting creative with maroon color placement. (Don't worry if edges are uneven; you will soon outline the shapes in gold glitter striper polish.) Apply to all nails and allow to dry, then apply a second coat if denser color coverage is needed and allow to dry.

Step 3

Apply pink polish wherever you like, in complementary angular shapes as you did with the maroon polish. Apply to all nails and allow to dry.

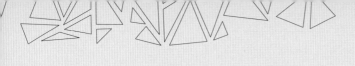

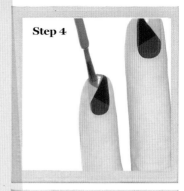

Step 4

Repeat step 3, applying blue polish in complementary angular shapes, and allow to dry.

Step 5

With the gold glitter striper polish, paint lines where the different colors meet, applying light, even strokes. Repeat until you are happy with the density of the glitter, allowing time to dry in between coats.

Step 6

When dry, apply clear top coat and allow the completed look to dry.

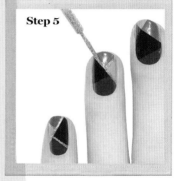

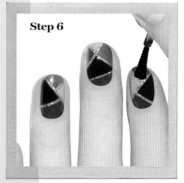

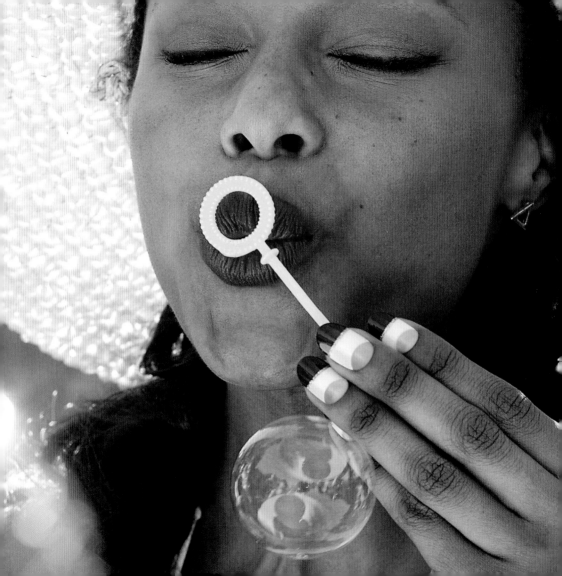

Nautical

Navy and cream keep it classy, while a gold band lends a touch of glamour. Take this look to the seaside, or pair with winter whites in the cooler months.

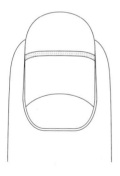

Tools:

- ☐ Clear base coat
- ☐ Paper reinforcements
- ☐ Tweezers
- ☐ Cream polish
- ☐ Clear top coat
- ☐ Angled-edge eyeliner brush (optional)

- ☐ Nail polish remover (optional)
- ☐ Paper towel (optional)
- ☐ Navy polish
- ☐ Gold glitter striper polish

(continued)

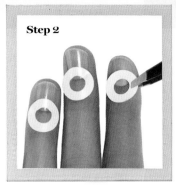

Step 2

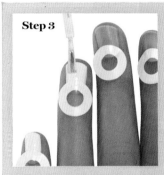

Step 3

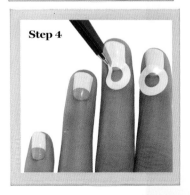

Step 4

Nautical Instructions

Step 1

Apply a clear base coat to all nails, which will strengthen the adhesion of the paper reinforcements. Allow to dry.

Step 2

Position a paper reinforcement on the bottom of each nail so the top of the reinforcement follows the line of the moon area (see Nail Anatomy, page 22). If your nail does not have a visible moon area, create one by placing the top of the paper reinforcement on the bottom of the nail, so that approximately one-third of the nail is covered. Press lightly so the paper reinforcement adheres to the nail, and use tweezers to press the reinforcement into the edges where the cuticle meets the nail.

Step 3

Paint the upper part of each nail with cream polish using upward strokes, swiping your brush across the top of the paper reinforcement and continuing to the top of the nail. Apply to all nails and allow to dry, then repeat with a second coat of cream polish.

Step 4

When polish is completely dry, use tweezers to remove the paper reinforcements, pulling carefully from one side to the other.

Step 5

If polish has leaked under the paper, leaving behind a jagged curved line, dip the angled-edge eyeliner brush into polish remover, press against a paper towel to soak up excess, and apply the bristles to the area for precise cleanup.

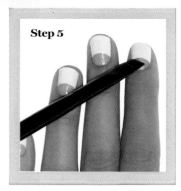

Step 6

Apply navy polish to the top half of all nails, using upward strokes from the midline to the tip of the nail. Allow to dry.

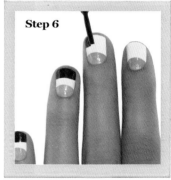

Step 7

With the gold glitter striper polish, paint the horizontal line where the cream section meets the navy section, starting from the edges of the nail and moving toward the center. Apply to all nails and allow to dry. Repeat this step until you have achieved the glitter density that you like, allowing time to dry after each coat.

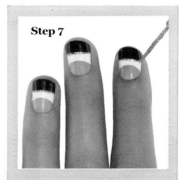

Step 8

When dry, apply clear top coat and allow the completed look to dry.

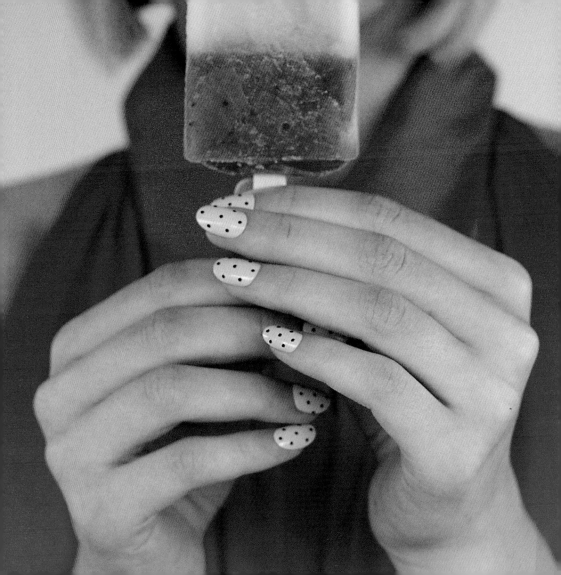

Glitter Studs

This flirty two-in-one look—sweet polka dots from afar, sexy studs up close—says there's more to you than meets the eye. Baby pink (or baby blue, as an alternative) provides an angelic backdrop to shimmering black hardware.

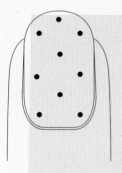

Tools:

- ☐ Black glitter
- ☐ Pink polish
- ☐ Clear top coat
- ☐ Disposable white plastic plate
- ☐ Double-sided dotting tool (or toothpick)

(continued)

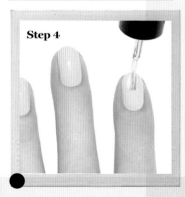

Glitter Studs Instructions

Step 1

Sprinkle a pinch of black glitter on your workspace for easy access.

Step 2

Apply one coat of pink polish to all nails and allow to dry.

Step 3

While allowing pink polish to dry, pour a pea-size drop of clear top coat on the plastic plate.

Step 4

Apply a second coat of pink to one nail and allow it to dry for 60 seconds. The slightly wet polish will act as an adhesive for the glitter.

Step 5

Dip the small end of the dotting tool into the puddle of clear top coat, then lightly touch it to a single piece of glitter. The glitter will adhere to the tip of the dotting tool for easy transfer to the nail. Position the dotting tool directly above the nail surface, wherever you want to apply the piece of glitter. Place the first piece of glitter in the center of the nail. Gently press the dotting tool to the nail and then lift off, leaving the glitter attached to the nail. (If using a toothpick instead of a dotting tool, slightly moisten the end and use it to pick up individual pieces of glitter, then apply to the nail as described above.)

Step 6

Repeat step 5, applying glitter above and below the center piece, leaving even amounts of space between each piece and creating a neat dotted line down the nail. Add dotted lines to either side, shifting the placement slightly to create a staggered design.

Step 7

Proceed to the next nail, repeating steps 4 to 6 until all nails are complete. If the puddle of top coat dries so that it does not adhere to the dotting tool, simply pour a fresh pea-size puddle.

Step 8

When dry, apply clear top coat and allow the completed look to dry.

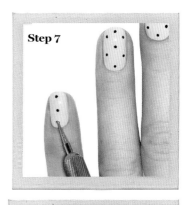

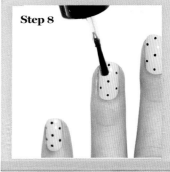

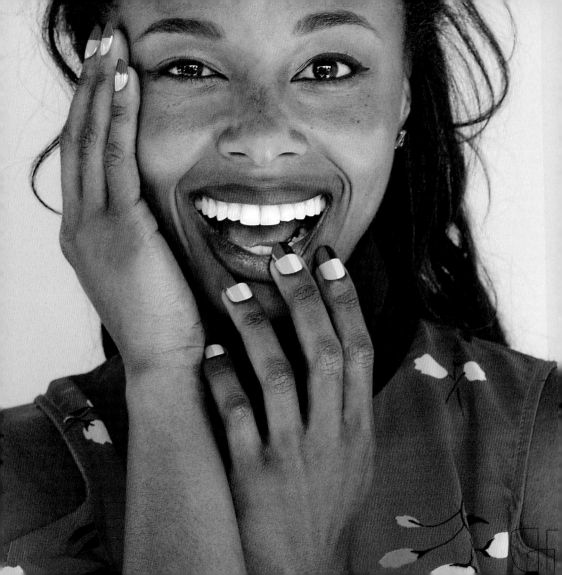

Cubic

Pretty and preppy, this look says the weekend is almost here. Have fun with color selection—go bright for high heat, soften up with pastels, or use black and white for a checkerboard effect.

Partner recommended.

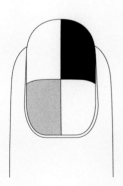

Tools:

☐ Light pink polish

☐ Light blue polish

☐ Red polish

☐ Black polish

☐ Clear top coat

(continued)

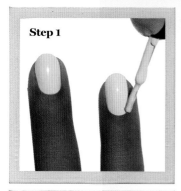

Step 1

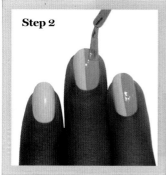

Step 2

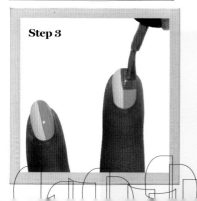

Step 3

Cubic Instructions

Note:

This look can feature any color assortment, but top color polishes should be opaque enough to cover the bottom color polishes.

Step 1

Apply two coats of light pink polish to all nails and allow to dry after each coat.

Step 2

Paint the right half of each nail with light blue polish, using a steady hand to create a smooth, even line from the bottom to the top of the nail. Allow to dry and apply a second coat if stronger coverage is needed.

Step 3

With red polish, paint the top right corner of each nail, using the flat edge of the brush to create straight lines. (Don't worry if you get polish outside the nail; you can clean up later.) Allow to dry, then apply a second coat if needed.

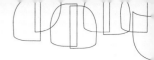

Step 4

With the black polish, paint the top left corner of each nail. Allow to dry, then apply a second coat if needed.

Step 5

When dry, apply clear top coat and allow the completed look to dry.

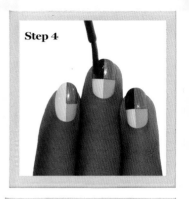

Step 4

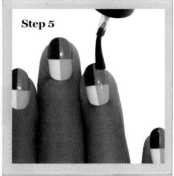

Step 5

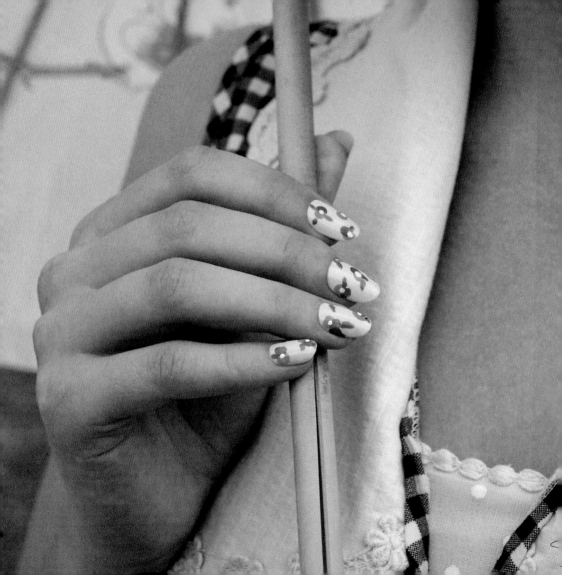

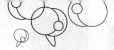

Abstract Floral

Overlapping dots and delicate lines give the impression of flowers in this girly, shabby-chic look. It's a bouquet that lasts and lasts, perfect for lunch with the ladies, outings to the flea market, or an afternoon tea party.

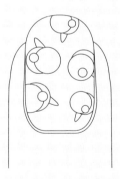

Tools:

- ☐ Pale peach polish
- ☐ Orange polish
- ☐ Disposable white plastic plate
- ☐ Cotton swab
- ☐ Pink polish
- ☐ White polish
- ☐ Double-sided dotting tool
- ☐ Green polish
- ☐ Clear top coat

(continued)

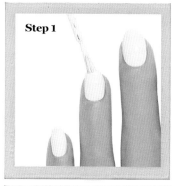

Abstract Floral Instructions

Step 1
Apply two coats of pale peach polish to all nails and allow to dry after each coat.

Step 2
Pour a dime-size puddle of orange polish on the plastic plate.

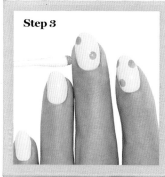

Step 3
Dip one end of a cotton swab into the orange puddle, generously coating the tip with polish. Add two or three orange dots to the nail. Dots should not be perfect circles, but rather soft, round shapes. Place dots at random, near the edges of the nail. Apply dots to each nail and allow to dry.

Step 4
Pour a dime-size puddle of pink polish on the plastic plate.

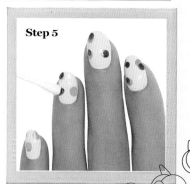

Step 5
Dip the other end of the cotton swab into the pink polish, generously coating the tip with polish. Add round dots that slightly overlap the orange dots. Pink dots can be the same size as the orange dots, or smaller, creating the look of abstract flower petals. Apply to all nails and allow to dry.

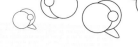

Step 6

Pour a pea-size puddle of white polish on the plastic plate.

Step 7

Dip the large end of the dotting tool into the white polish and apply to the point where the pink and orange dots overlap, creating a small white circle that suggests the center of the flower. Apply to all nails and allow to dry.

Step 8

To create green leaves, first make sure the green polish brush is not too heavily coated with polish. Reduce the amount of polish on the brush by wiping it along the inside opening of the polish bottle. This will also flatten the bristles into a wide but thin rectangle. Lightly touch the rectangular tip of the brush to the nail, extending from the pink and orange dots, wherever you would like leaves to appear. Apply to all nails and allow to dry.

Step 9

Apply clear top coat and allow the completed look to dry.

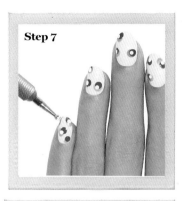

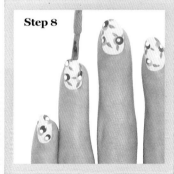

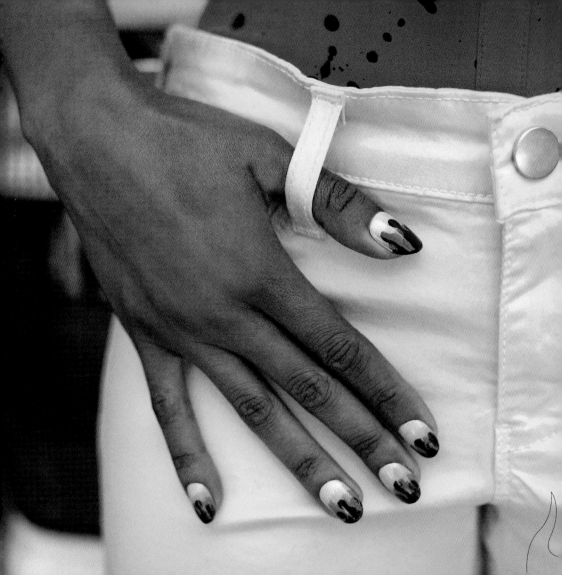

Flame

This fiery look will have your friends doing double takes. Seemingly advanced, the secret to this project is vertical streaks and a graphic silhouette. Wear at nighttime, on a camping trip, or on a cold winter's night—or whenever you're feeling fierce.

Partner recommended.

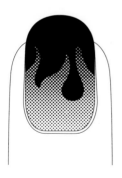

Tools:

- ☐ Yellow polish
- ☐ Orange polish
- ☐ Red polish
- ☐ Black striper polish
- ☐ Clear top coat

(continued)

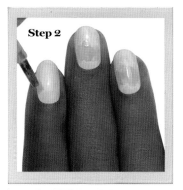

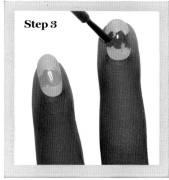

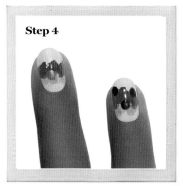

Flame Instructions

Step 1

Apply two coats of yellow polish to all nails and allow to dry after each coat.

Step 2

With the orange polish, paint three vertical streaks above the cuticle, leaving a ragged horizontal strip of yellow at the bottom of the nail. Apply to all nails and allow to dry.

Step 3

With the red polish, paint three vertical streaks overlapping the top of the orange streaks, leaving a ragged strip of orange between the red and the yellow. Apply to all nails and allow to dry.

Step 4

With the black striper polish, paint a small black circle in the center of the nail and two smaller circles, one on either side and close to the edge of the nail.

Step 5

Connect the black circles by painting curves with the striper polish, creating flame outlines. Fill in the black space at the top of the nail. Apply to all nails.

Step 6

When dry, apply a second coat of black to the top of all nails, carefully preserving the flame outlines.

Step 7

When dry, apply clear top coat and allow the completed look to dry.

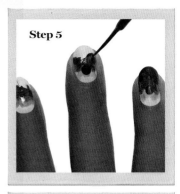

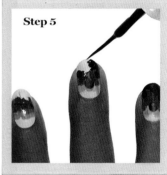

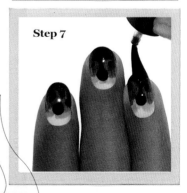

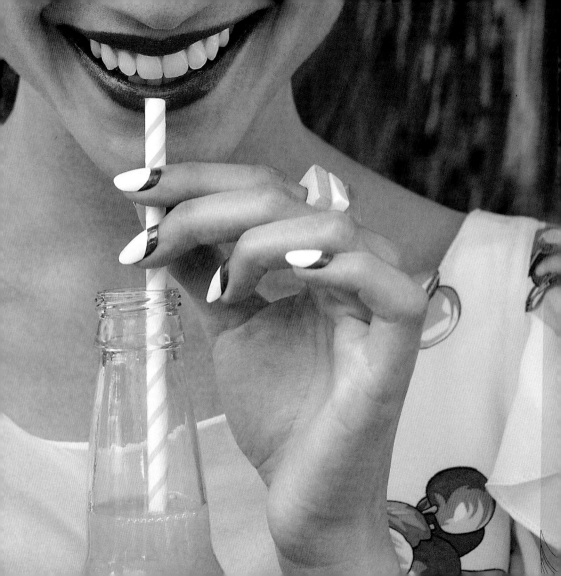

Triple Eclipse

This lunar look features warm, muted colors and bohemian, 1970s flair. Build an outfit with aviator sunglasses, knee-high boots, and a leather-fringed purse. Or change up the colors—three shades of blue make an icy cool trio, while amber, orange, and yellow will bring on a sunrise.

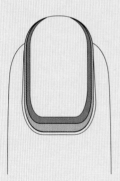

Tools:

☐ Red polish

☐ Green polish

☐ Cream polish

☐ Clear top coat

(continued)

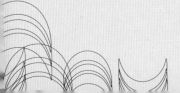

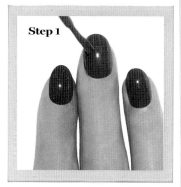

Triple Eclipse Instructions

Note:

Make sure the cream polish has a high opacity for dense color coverage. If cream opacity is too low, use a different color that will sufficiently cover the underlying green color.

Step 1

Apply one coat of red polish to all nails and allow to dry.

Step 2

With green polish, paint an upward-facing curved line above the bottom edge of each nail, echoing the line of the cuticle and leaving a curved rim of red at the bottom of the nail. Fill in the top of each nail with green polish. Allow to dry.

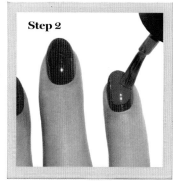

Step 3

Repeat step 2 with the cream polish, leaving a green curve that is roughly the same width as the orange curve. Allow to dry, then apply a second coat.

Step 4

When dry, apply clear top coat and allow the completed look to dry.

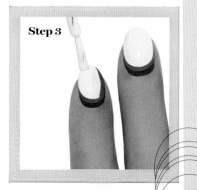

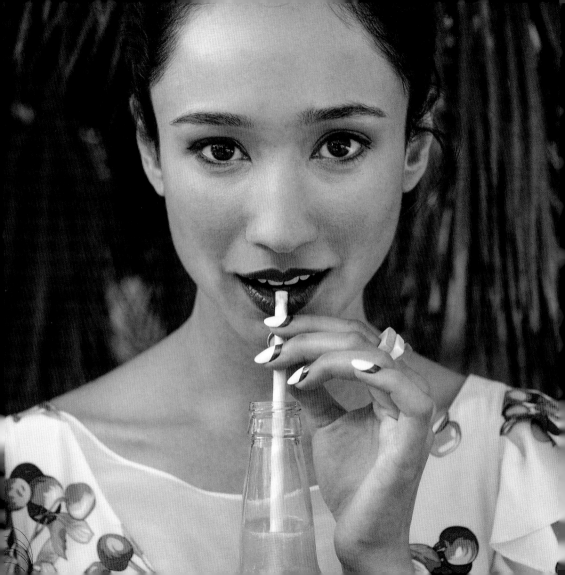

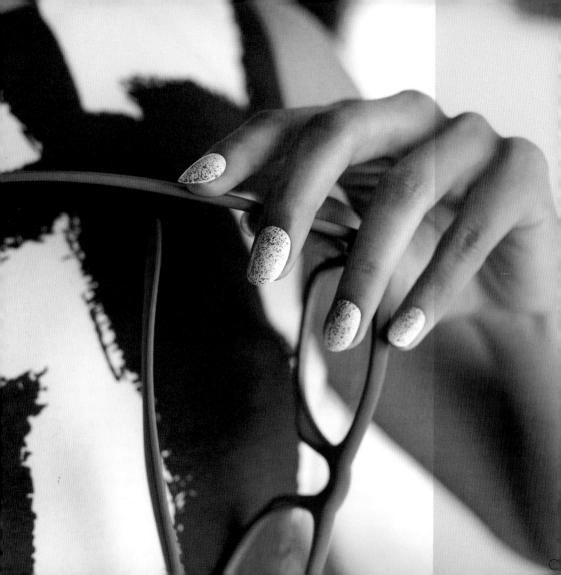

Spray Paint

Step up your street style with nail graffiti, featuring smears, splatters, and spray. Nails are a blank canvas in this artsy look, which is as exciting to create as it is to wear.

Partner recommended.

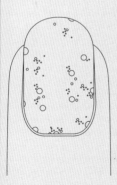

Tools:

- ☐ Newspaper
- ☐ White polish
- ☐ Purple polish
- ☐ Disposable white plastic plate
- ☐ Rubber gloves

- ☐ Toothbrush
- ☐ Clear top coat
- ☐ Nail polish remover
- ☐ Cotton swabs

(continued)

Spray Paint Instructions

Notes:

To avoid a mess on your hands, you can apply the design to a set of false nails.

Practice your spray technique on the plastic plate before applying it to the nail—it might take a few times to get it just right.

If your toothbrush absorbs too much polish, resulting in a weak spray, simply use the toothbrush like a paint-brush, pressing it into the nail to create a mottled, marbled effect.

Step 1

Spread a piece of newspaper across your work-space for extra protection, as things are about to get messy!

Step 2

Apply two coats of white polish to all nails and allow to dry after each coat.

Step 3

Place a dime-size puddle of purple nail polish on the plastic plate. Pour more as needed throughout the project.

Step 4

Put a rubber glove on your working hand (the one you are not painting).

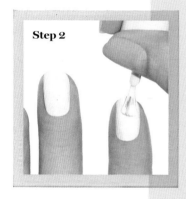

Step 2

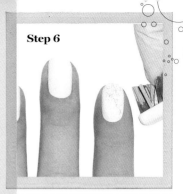

Step 5

Dip the uppermost bristles of the toothbrush in the puddle of purple polish, coating the bristles thoroughly.

Step 6

Flatten your ungloved hand on your work surface. With your gloved hand, grip the toothbrush so your pointer finger has access to the bristles, and position the brush over the nail you want to spray. Press down the bristles with your pointer finger and then release them, letting paint spray across the nail. Apply to all nails, and don't worry about making a mess on your workspace or hands; you can clean up later. Allow to dry.

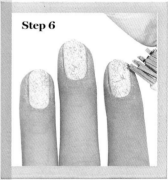

Step 7

Apply clear top coat to the completed nails and allow 20 minutes to dry.

Step 8

While nails are drying, use a cotton swab to apply nail polish remover to the cuticle and anywhere on the fingers where polish might have sprayed.

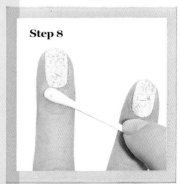

Step 9

When dry, repeat steps 4 to 8, applying purple spray and clear top coat to the nails of the other hand, and allow to dry.

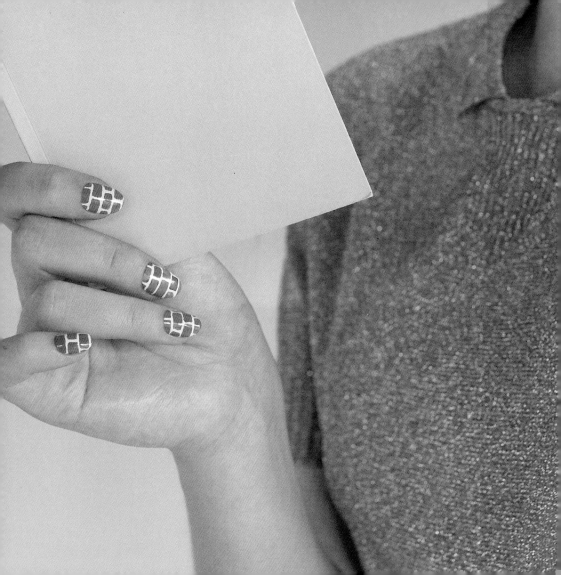

Brick

This crafty look will inspire you to build and create, one brick at a time. Speckled red from afar, a closer look reveals an intricate grid that is both pretty and practical, turning heads and playing tricks on the eye.

Partner recommended.

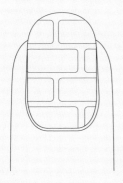

Tools:

☐ Cream polish

☐ Brick red
striper polish

☐ Clear top coat

(continued)

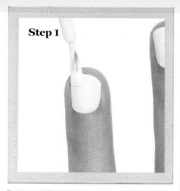

Brick Instructions

Step 1

Apply two coats of cream polish to all nails and allow to dry after each coat.

Step 2

With the brick red striper polish, paint two equal-size horizontal rectangles at the midline of the nail.

Step 3

Directly above and below the midline, paint new lines of rectangles—three per row or one long rectangle—to create a staggered look.

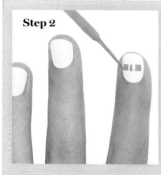

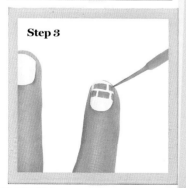

Step 4

Continue adding staggered rows of rectangles until the nail is covered with brick pattern.

Step 5

Proceed to the next nail and continue until all nails feature the design.

Step 6

When dry, apply clear top coat and allow the completed look to dry.

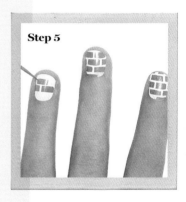

Step 5

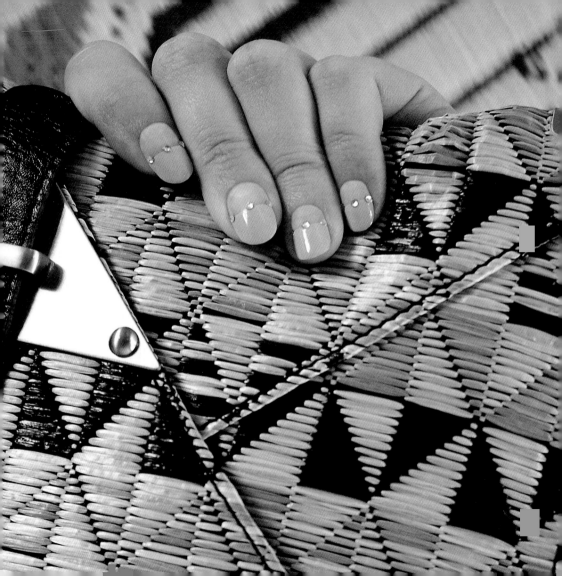

Half Nail with Crystals

Who needs glass slippers when you have Cinderella nails? Sweet and feminine, this look is pure magic, combining the beauty of the natural nail with the polish of a princess.

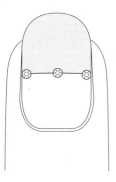

Tools:

- ☐ 30 nail crystals
- ☐ Scissors
- ☐ Sticky tape
- ☐ Tweezers
- ☐ Baby blue polish
- ☐ Clear top coat
- ☐ Disposable white plastic plate

- ☐ Nail glue
- ☐ Double-sided dotting tool (optional)

(continued)

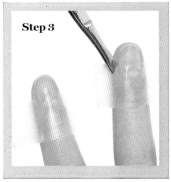

Step 3

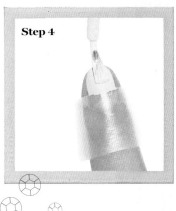

Step 4

Half Nail with Crystals Instructions

Note:

Nail glue is a strong adhesive, so apply with care and read instructions thoroughly before use.

Step 1

Sprinkle crystals on your workspace for easy access, and make sure each crystal lies flat on its underside.

Step 2

Cut ten pieces of tape that are each slightly longer than the width of each nail. Lightly stick pieces to the edge of a table surface until needed.

Step 3

With tweezers, place a piece of tape horizontally across the middle of each nail. Press firmly, and use tweezers to press tape into the edges where the nail meets the cuticle.

Step 4

Paint the top half of each nail with baby blue polish using upward strokes. Allow to dry, then repeat with a second coat.

Step 5

When nails are completely dry, use tweezers to remove the tape, pulling gently from left to right.

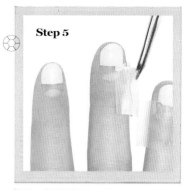
Step 5

Step 6

If using a dotting tool to apply crystals, pour a pea-size drop of clear top coat on the plastic plate.

Step 7

Apply a tiny drop of nail glue to the center of one nail, on the midline where the baby blue polish meets the natural-colored nail.

Step 8

Dip the small end of the dotting tool into the puddle of clear top coat, then lightly touch it to the top of a single crystal. The crystal will adhere to the tip of the dotting tool for easy transfer to the nail. Position the dotting tool directly above the nail, gently placing the crystal on top of the glue drop. (If you don't have a dotting tool, use tweezers to transfer the crystals.)

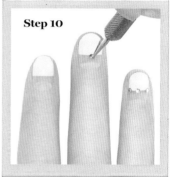
Step 10

Step 9

Repeat steps 7 and 8, applying nail glue and crystals to the right and left of the center crystal, creating a line of three crystals along the midline of the nail.

Step 10

Apply crystals to all nails and allow the glue to dry thoroughly.

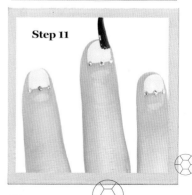
Step 11

Step 11

Apply clear top coat, painting the entire surface of each nail, and allow the completed look to dry.

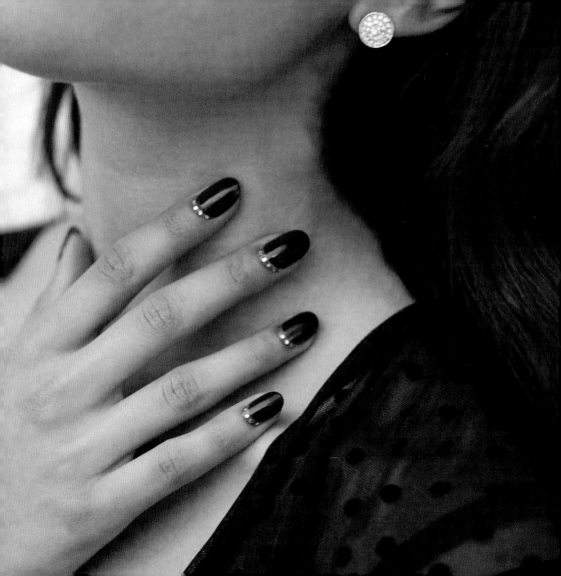

Studded Eclipse

Give your nails the royal treatment with layered purple and a glitter lining. Fancy and fun, this look is Hollywood after dark. Wear with lipstick and furs, or dress it down with dark denim.

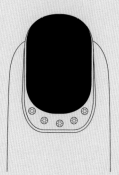

Tools:

☐ Gold glitter

☐ Two shades of purple polish (one light, one dark)

☐ Clear top coat

☐ Disposable white plastic plate

☐ Double-sided dotting tool (or toothpick)

(continued)

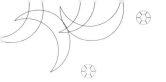

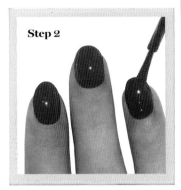

Step 2

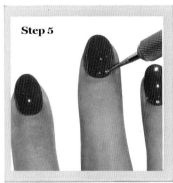

Step 5

Studded Eclipse Instructions

Step 1
Sprinkle a pinch of gold glitter on your workspace for easy access.

Step 2
Apply one coat of light purple polish to all nails and allow to dry.

Step 3
If using a dotting tool to apply glitter, pour a pea-size puddle of clear top coat on the plastic plate.

Step 4
Apply a second coat of light purple polish to the bottom half of one nail and allow to dry for 60 seconds. The slightly wet polish will act as an adhesive for the glitter.

Step 5
Lightly dip the small end of the dotting tool into the puddle of clear top coat, then lightly touch it to a single piece of glitter. The glitter will adhere to the tip of the dotting tool for easy transfer to the nail. Position the dotting tool directly above the nail surface at the bottom center of the nail. Gently press the dotting tool to the nail and then lift off, leaving the glitter attached to the nail. (If using a

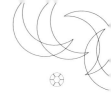

toothpick instead of a dotting tool, slightly moisten the end and use it to pick up individual pieces of glitter, then apply to the nail as described.)

Step 6

Repeat step 5, adding pieces of glitter to the right and left of the center piece—echoing the line of the cuticle—until there are five to seven pieces of glitter in a row along the bottom curve of the nail. (Leave plenty of room around each piece so the underlying shade of purple is visible.)

Step 7

Repeat steps 4 to 6, applying glitter to each nail, and allow to dry. If the puddle of top coat dries, simply pour a fresh pea-size puddle.

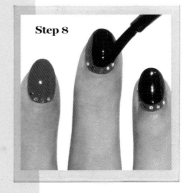

Step 8

Step 8

With dark purple polish, paint an upward-facing curved line above the bottom edge of each nail, echoing the line of glitter and leaving a wide curved rim of light purple at the bottom of each nail. Fill in the top of each nail with dark purple polish. Allow to dry, and apply a second coat if needed.

Step 9

When dry, apply a clear top coat, covering each nail completely, and allow the finished look to dry.

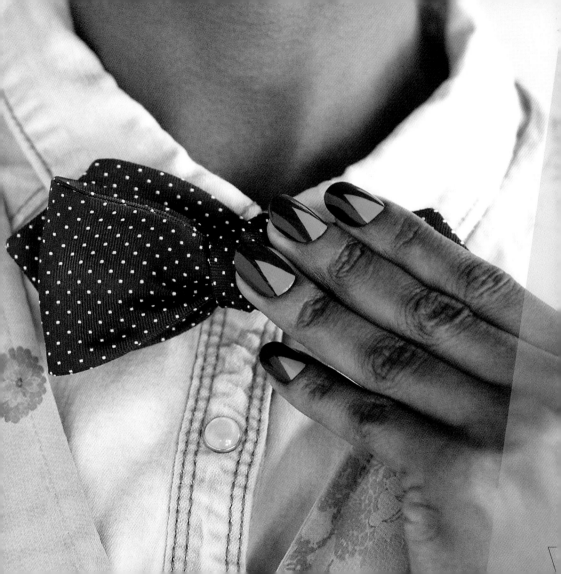

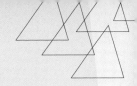

Pyramid Point

This sleek, two-toned look oozes confidence and style and is fabulous with any polish color pairing. Try pastels for subtle geometry, or neons to really make your point.

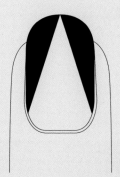

Tools:

- ☐ Turquoise polish
- ☐ Dark blue polish
- ☐ Clear top coat

(continued)

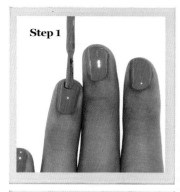

Step 1

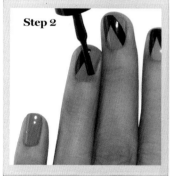

Step 2

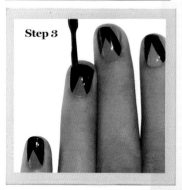

Step 3

Pyramid Point Instructions

Step 1

Apply two coats of turquoise polish to all nails and allow to dry after each coat.

Step 2

With dark blue polish, create two long strokes from the bottom corners of the nail to the center tip, leaving a turquoise triangle in the middle.

Step 3

Fill in outer areas of the triangle with dark blue polish. Apply to all nails and allow to dry.

Step 4

Apply a second coat of dark blue to all nails, carefully preserving the straight lines of the triangle.

Step 5

When dry, apply clear top coat and allow the completed look to dry.

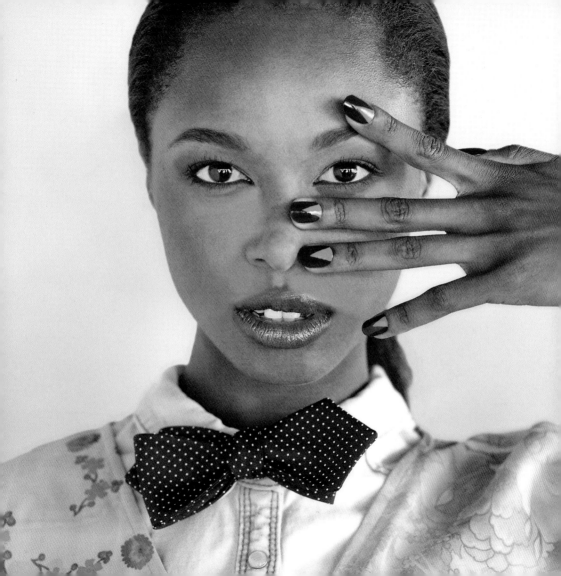

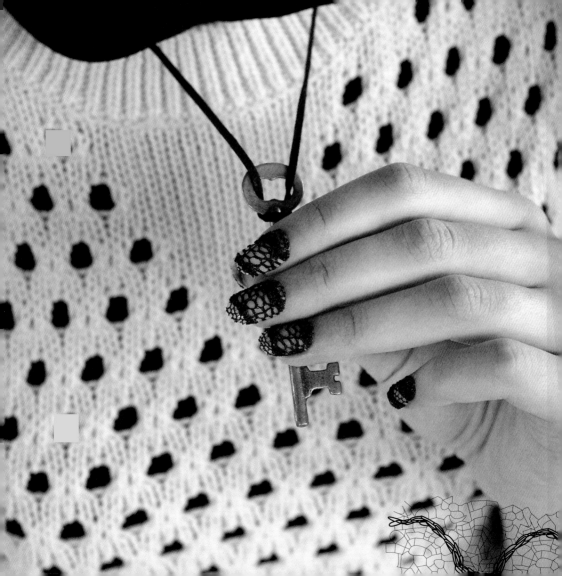

Lace

Dress up your nails with this fun, textured style. Wear it with fingerless gloves for an edgy look, or use white lace for a dainty design.

Partner recommended.

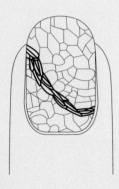

Tools:

- ☐ Scissors
- ☐ Black lace
- ☐ Clear top coat
- ☐ Tweezers
- ☐ Damp paper towel

(continued)

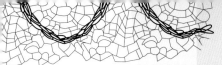

Lace Instructions

Step 1

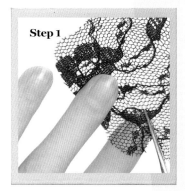

Cut pieces of lace for each nail by placing the nail under the lace and carefully cutting an outline of the nail. (It's okay if pieces are longer than your nails—you will trim the tips after they have been adhered to the nail.) Spread out the lace pieces on your workspace in the order in which they will appear on your nails.

Step 2

Apply one layer of clear top coat to one nail and do not allow it to dry. The wet top coat will act as an adhesive for the lace.

Step 3

Using tweezers, place the corresponding piece of lace on the nail.

Step 4

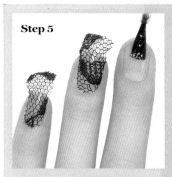

Moisten a finger on the damp paper towel and press the lace to the nail, positioning it neatly. Use tweezers to stretch the lace to the edges of the nail.

Step 5

Proceed to the next nail, repeating steps 2 to 4, and continue the design until all nails on one hand are adorned with lace. Allow to dry.

equires a large amount of clear base coat.
ur bottle is at least one quarter full.

bats of blue polish to all nails and allow
each coat.

ic plate, pour a puddle of clear base
the size of a nickel. Nearby, pour a
p of neon pink polish. Dip the tip of
edge eyeliner brush into the neon
x neon pink into the base coat pud-
a blend that is pink-tinted but mostly

gled-edge eyeliner brush, apply a thin
blended polish to the top two-thirds of
ting near the bottom of the nail and
the tip. Apply to all ten nails and

ic plate, create a new nickel-size pud-
base coat, and a new pea-size pud-
pink polish. With the angled-edge
h, mix neon pink into the base coat

Step 6

With scissors, carefully trim the top edge of all lace
pieces so they neatly align with the tips of your
nails.

Step 7

Apply top coat to the lace-covered nails and allow
to dry.

Step 8

Repeat steps 2 to 7, applying lace and top coat to
the nails on the other hand.

Step 9

When dry, apply a second layer of top coat to all
nails, and allow the finished look to dry.

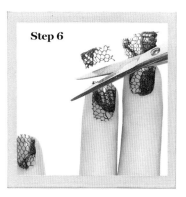

Step 6

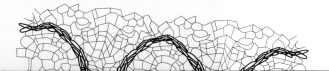

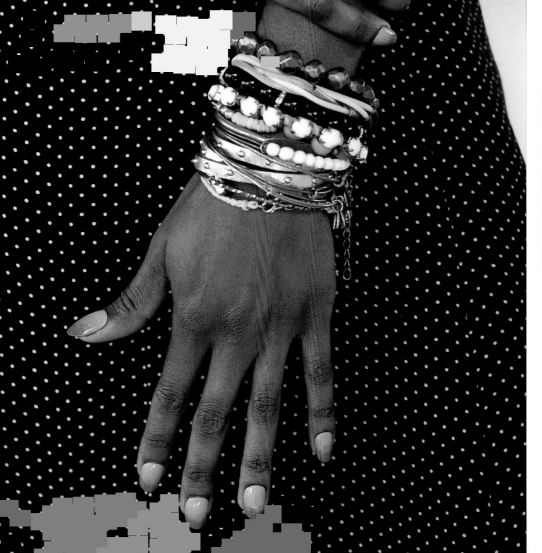

Electric

Note:

*This project ᵣ
Make sure yₒ*

Step 1

Apply two c
to dry after

Step 2

On the plas
coat about
pea-size dr
the angleᵈ
pink and m
dle, creatin
translucent

Step 3

Using the aᵣ
coat of the
the nail, sta
continuing ᵗ
allow to dry

Step 4

On the plas
dle of fresh
dle of neon
eyeliner brᵤ

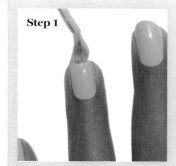

Step 1

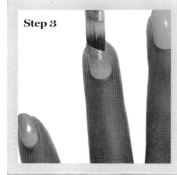

Step 3

(using twice as much pink as used in step 2) and blend together. The resulting color should still be translucent but the pink tint should be twice as strong.

Step 5

Apply a thin coat of the blended polish to the top half of all nails and allow to dry.

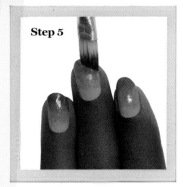

Step 6

Create new puddles of base coat and neon pink polish on the plastic plate, the same size as previously described. Blend neon pink polish into the base coat, once again doubling the amount of pink polish. The resulting color should be predominantly neon pink but still translucent. Apply to the top third of each nail and allow to dry.

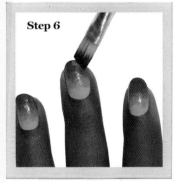

Step 7

Apply pure, unblended neon pink polish to the tip of each nail.

Step 8

When dry, apply clear top coat and allow the completed look to dry.

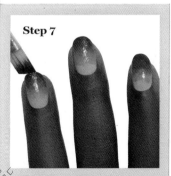

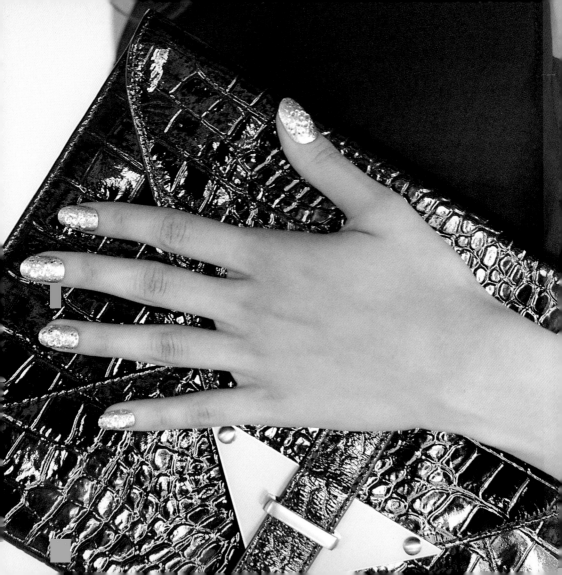

Jewel-Encrusted

Channel an Egyptian queen with this gilded, glitzy look. Super fun to make and sure to light up a room, it is also versatile and wardrobe-friendly. Pair it with a cocktail dress or a simple black tee for equally glam results.

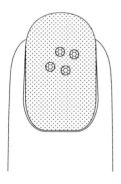

Tools:

- [ ] Gold glitter
- [ ] 30 to 40 nail crystals (approximately 3 to 4 per nail)
- [ ] Gold polish
- [ ] Gold glitter polish
- [ ] Clear top coat

- [ ] Disposable white plastic plate
- [ ] Double-sided dotting tool (or toothpick and tweezers)
- [ ] Nail glue

(continued)

Jewel-Encrusted Instructions

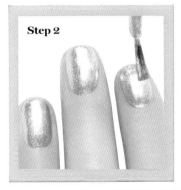

Step 2

Note:

Nail glue is a strong adhesive, so apply with care and read instructions thoroughly before use.

Step 1

Sprinkle a pinch of glitter and arrange crystals flat-side down on your workspace.

Step 2

Apply two coats of gold polish to all nails, then one coat of gold glitter polish, and allow to dry after each coat.

Step 3

Pour a pea-size puddle of clear top coat on the plastic plate.

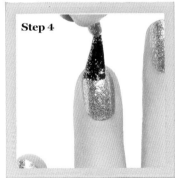

Step 4

Step 4

Apply a second coat of gold glitter polish to one nail and don't allow it to dry. The wet polish will act as an adhesive for the glitter.

Step 5

Dip the small end of the dotting tool into the puddle of top coat, then lightly touch it to a piece of glitter. The glitter will adhere to the tip of the dotting tool. Position the dotting tool directly above the nail surface, wherever you want to apply the piece of glitter. Gently press the dotting tool to the nail and then lift off, leaving the glitter attached to

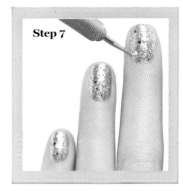
Step 7

the nail. (If using a toothpick instead of a dotting tool, slightly moisten the end and use it to pick up individual pieces of glitter, then apply to the nail as described.)

Step 6

Leaving the center area of the nail empty, apply glitter pieces all around the nail—as many as you like.

Step 7

Repeat steps 4 to 6 for each nail and allow to dry.

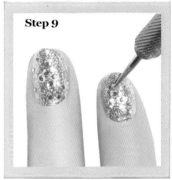
Step 9

Step 8

Place a tiny drop of glue on the center of the nail, then transfer a crystal to the glue using the dotting tool, as described in step 5. (If you don't have a dotting tool, use tweezers.) Continue adding glue and crystals to the nail center to create a cluster.

Step 9

Repeat step 8, adding a cluster to each nail, and allow glue to dry.

Step 10

Apply clear top coat and allow the completed look to dry.

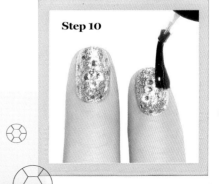
Step 10

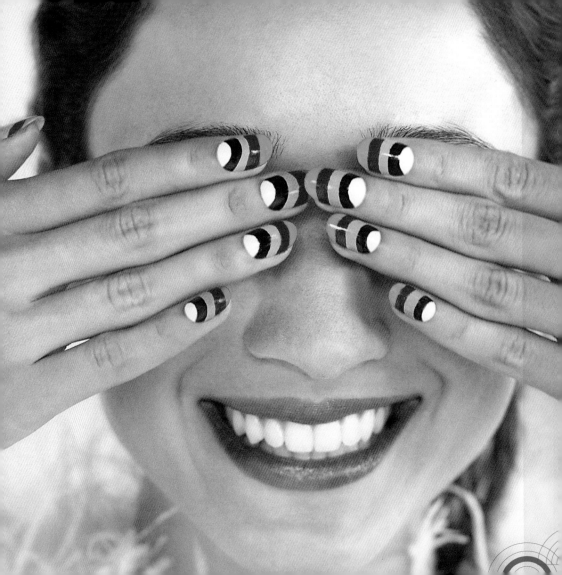

Multistripe

Featuring creative line placement, this project is great for flexing your new nail art skills. Woven stripes offer candy-colored fun—or, apply neon polishes for a hypnotic effect.

Partner recommended.

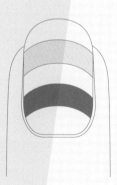

Tools:

- ☐ Yellow polish
- ☐ Pink polish
- ☐ Turquoise polish
- ☐ Black striper polish
- ☐ Red striper polish
- ☐ Clear top coat

(continued)

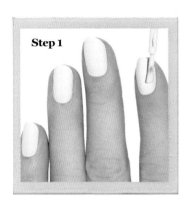

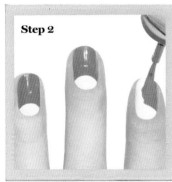

Multistripe Instructions

Note:

Make every nail look different by alternating color placement on each nail. Or, turn stripes upside down on every other nail for topsy-turvy rainbows.

Step 1

Apply two coats of yellow polish to all nails and allow time to dry after each coat.

Step 2

With pink polish, paint around the moon area (see Nail Anatomy, page 22) by first painting a curve that rises approximately one third from the bottom of each nail. Don't worry if the curved edge is not perfect—you will soon cover this border with another color. Fill in the area above the curve with pink polish. Allow to dry, then apply a second coat of pink if stronger coverage is needed.

Step 3

When pink polish is dry, paint the top one-third of each nail with turquoise polish, creating a curved shape that echoes the shape of the moon area. As in the previous step, don't worry if the curved edge is not perfect—you will soon cover this border with another color. Allow to dry, then repeat with a second coat of turquoise polish.

Step 4

When nails are completely dry, use the black striper polish to paint a curved black line between the pink and the yellow layers, as thick or as thin as you want it. Apply to all nails and allow to dry, then apply a second coat if needed.

Step 5

When nails are completely dry, use the red striper polish to paint a curved red line between the pink and turquoise layers, as thick or as thin as you want it. Apply to all nails and allow to dry, then repeat with a second coat if needed.

Step 6

When dry, apply clear top coat and allow the completed look to dry.

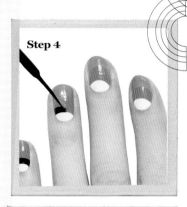

Step 4

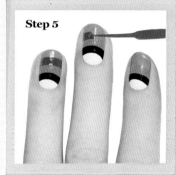

Step 5

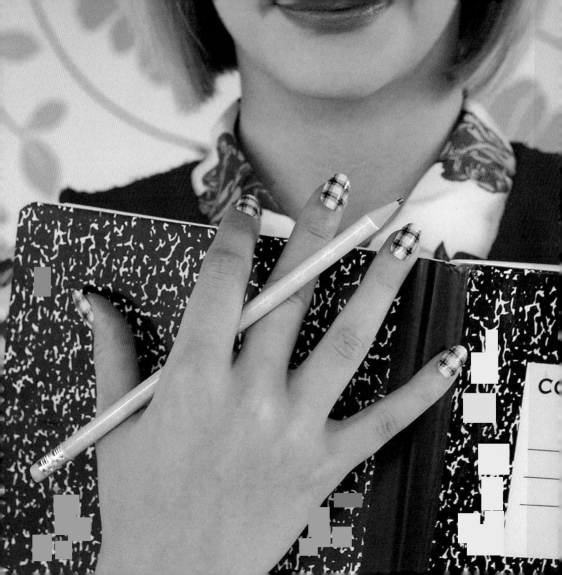

Plaid

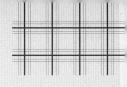

Bring out your inner schoolgirl with this traditional motif, perfect for playing hooky or burying yourself in a book. And don't worry about curfew—plaid is playful round-the-clock!

Partner recommended.

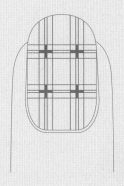

Tools:

- ☐ Yellow polish
- ☐ Light gray polish
- ☐ Dark gray striper polish
- ☐ Black striper polish
- ☐ Clear top coat

    (continued)

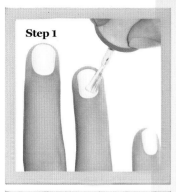

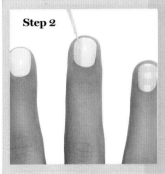

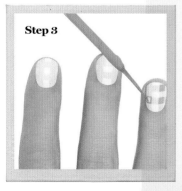

Plaid Instructions

Step 1

Apply two coats of yellow polish to all nails and allow to dry after each coat.

Step 2

With the light gray polish, paint two vertical lines and two horizontal lines, creating an evenly spaced grid. Apply to all nails and allow to dry.

Step 3

With the dark gray striper polish, fill in the squares where the vertical and horizontal lines intersect. Apply to all nails and allow to dry.

Lace

Dress up your nails with this fun, textured style. Wear it with fingerless gloves for an edgy look, or use white lace for a dainty design.

Partner recommended.

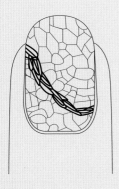

Tools:

☐ Scissors

☐ Black lace

☐ Clear top coat

☐ Tweezers

☐ Damp paper towel

(continued)

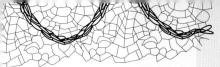

Lace Instructions

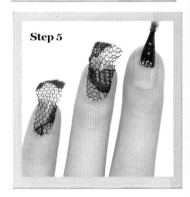

Step 1

Cut pieces of lace for each nail by placing the nail under the lace and carefully cutting an outline of the nail. (It's okay if pieces are longer than your nails—you will trim the tips after they have been adhered to the nail.) Spread out the lace pieces on your workspace in the order in which they will appear on your nails.

Step 2

Apply one layer of clear top coat to one nail and do not allow it to dry. The wet top coat will act as an adhesive for the lace.

Step 3

Using tweezers, place the corresponding piece of lace on the nail.

Step 4

Moisten a finger on the damp paper towel and press the lace to the nail, positioning it neatly. Use tweezers to stretch the lace to the edges of the nail.

Step 5

Proceed to the next nail, repeating steps 2 to 4, and continue the design until all nails on one hand are adorned with lace. Allow to dry.

Step 6

With scissors, carefully trim the top edge of all lace pieces so they neatly align with the tips of your nails.

Step 7

Apply top coat to the lace-covered nails and allow to dry.

Step 8

Repeat steps 2 to 7, applying lace and top coat to the nails on the other hand.

Step 9

When dry, apply a second layer of top coat to all nails, and allow the finished look to dry.

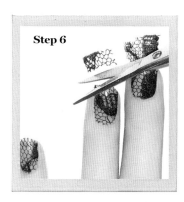

Step 6

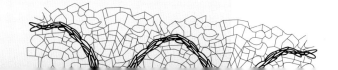

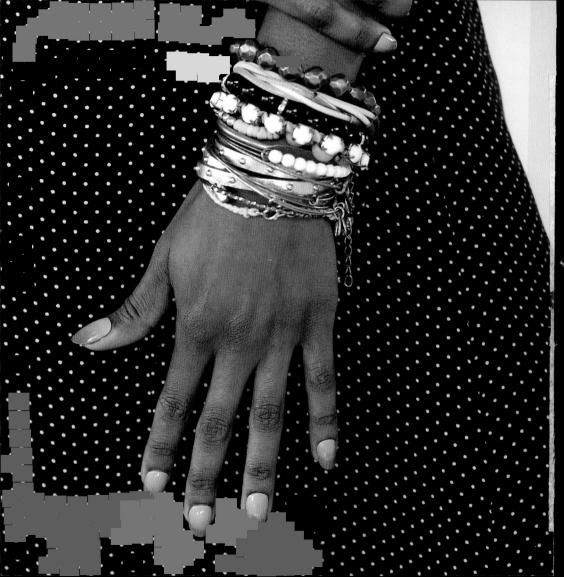

Electric Fade

Sporty and bold, the Electric Fade is a flashback to the 1980s—think pop ballads and Miami sunsets—when high-gloss nails were the finishing touch to any outfit. Modernize the look with stark white jeans and a bright tee, or stacked statement jewelry.

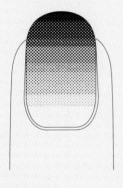

Tools:

- ☐ Light blue polish
- ☐ Disposable white plastic plate
- ☐ Clear base coat
- ☐ Neon pink polish
- ☐ Angled-edge eyeliner brush
- ☐ Clear top coat

(continued)

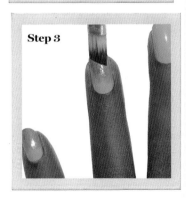

Step 1

Step 3

Electric Fade Instructions

Note:

This project requires a large amount of clear base coat. Make sure your bottle is at least one quarter full.

Step 1

Apply two coats of blue polish to all nails and allow to dry after each coat.

Step 2

On the plastic plate, pour a puddle of clear base coat about the size of a nickel. Nearby, pour a pea-size drop of neon pink polish. Dip the tip of the angled-edge eyeliner brush into the neon pink and mix neon pink into the base coat puddle, creating a blend that is pink-tinted but mostly translucent.

Step 3

Using the angled-edge eyeliner brush, apply a thin coat of the blended polish to the top two-thirds of the nail, starting near the bottom of the nail and continuing to the tip. Apply to all ten nails and allow to dry.

Step 4

On the plastic plate, create a new nickel-size puddle of fresh base coat, and a new pea-size puddle of neon pink polish. With the angled-edge eyeliner brush, mix neon pink into the base coat

Jewel-Encrusted

Channel an Egyptian queen with this gilded, glitzy look. Super fun to make and sure to light up a room, it is also versatile and wardrobe-friendly. Pair it with a cocktail dress or a simple black tee for equally glam results.

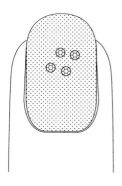

Tools:

- ☐ Gold glitter
- ☐ 30 to 40 nail crystals (approximately 3 to 4 per nail)
- ☐ Gold polish
- ☐ Gold glitter polish
- ☐ Clear top coat
- ☐ Disposable white plastic plate
- ☐ Double-sided dotting tool (or toothpick and tweezers)
- ☐ Nail glue

(continued)

Jewel-Encrusted Instructions

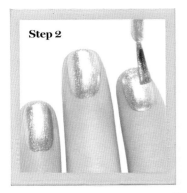

Step 2

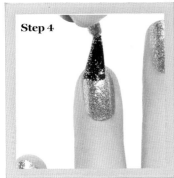

Step 4

Note:

Nail glue is a strong adhesive, so apply with care and read instructions thoroughly before use.

Step 1

Sprinkle a pinch of glitter and arrange crystals flat-side down on your workspace.

Step 2

Apply two coats of gold polish to all nails, then one coat of gold glitter polish, and allow to dry after each coat.

Step 3

Pour a pea-size puddle of clear top coat on the plastic plate.

Step 4

Apply a second coat of gold glitter polish to one nail and don't allow it to dry. The wet polish will act as an adhesive for the glitter.

Step 5

Dip the small end of the dotting tool into the puddle of top coat, then lightly touch it to a piece of glitter. The glitter will adhere to the tip of the dotting tool. Position the dotting tool directly above the nail surface, wherever you want to apply the piece of glitter. Gently press the dotting tool to the nail and then lift off, leaving the glitter attached to

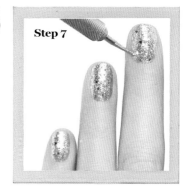

Step 7

the nail. (If using a toothpick instead of a dotting tool, slightly moisten the end and use it to pick up individual pieces of glitter, then apply to the nail as described.)

Step 6

Leaving the center area of the nail empty, apply glitter pieces all around the nail—as many as you like.

Step 7

Repeat steps 4 to 6 for each nail and allow to dry.

Step 8

Place a tiny drop of glue on the center of the nail, then transfer a crystal to the glue using the dotting tool, as described in step 5. (If you don't have a dotting tool, use tweezers.) Continue adding glue and crystals to the nail center to create a cluster.

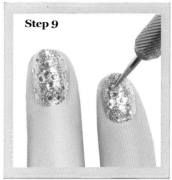

Step 9

Step 9

Repeat step 8, adding a cluster to each nail, and allow glue to dry.

Step 10

Apply clear top coat and allow the completed look to dry.

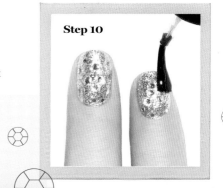

Step 10

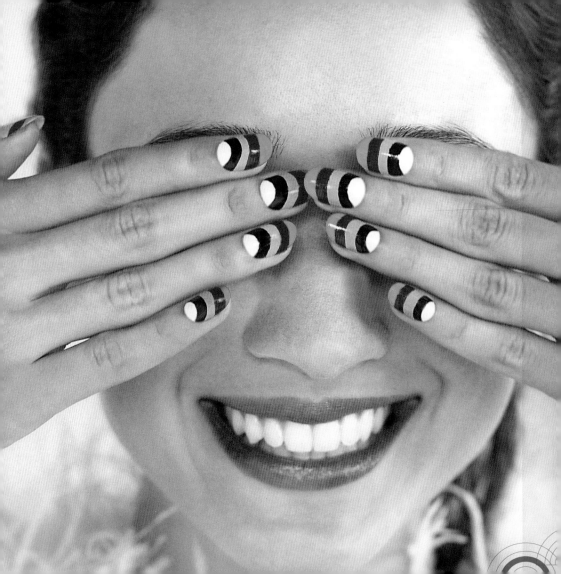

(using twice as much pink as used in step 2) and blend together. The resulting color should still be translucent but the pink tint should be twice as strong.

Step 5

Apply a thin coat of the blended polish to the top half of all nails and allow to dry.

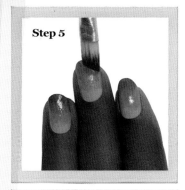

Step 6

Create new puddles of base coat and neon pink polish on the plastic plate, the same size as previously described. Blend neon pink polish into the base coat, once again doubling the amount of pink polish. The resulting color should be predominantly neon pink but still translucent. Apply to the top third of each nail and allow to dry.

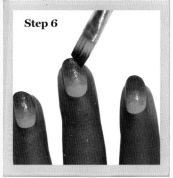

Step 7

Apply pure, unblended neon pink polish to the tip of each nail.

Step 8

When dry, apply clear top coat and allow the completed look to dry.

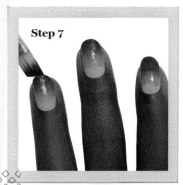

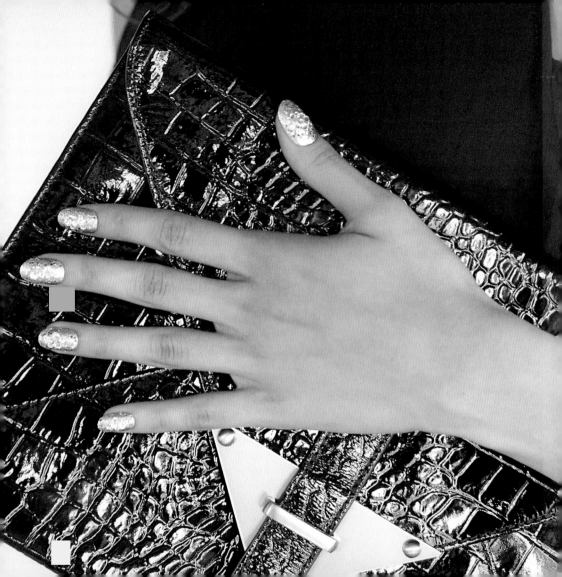

Multistripe

Featuring creative line placement, this project is great for flexing your new nail art skills. Woven stripes offer candy-colored fun—or, apply neon polishes for a hypnotic effect.

Partner recommended.

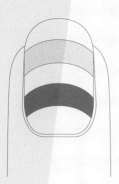

Tools:

☐ Yellow polish

☐ Pink polish

☐ Turquoise polish

☐ Black striper polish

☐ Red striper polish

☐ Clear top coat

(continued)

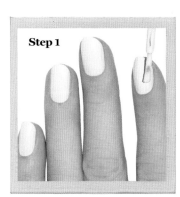

Step 1

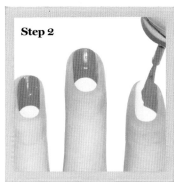

Step 2

Multistripe Instructions

Note:

Make every nail look different by alternating color place-ment on each nail. Or, turn stripes upside down on every other nail for topsy-turvy rainbows.

Step 1

Apply two coats of yellow polish to all nails and allow time to dry after each coat.

Step 2

With pink polish, paint around the moon area (see Nail Anatomy, page 22) by first painting a curve that rises approximately one third from the bottom of each nail. Don't worry if the curved edge is not perfect—you will soon cover this border with another color. Fill in the area above the curve with pink polish. Allow to dry, then apply a second coat of pink if stronger coverage is needed.

Step 3

When pink polish is dry, paint the top one-third of each nail with turquoise polish, creating a curved shape that echoes the shape of the moon area. As in the previous step, don't worry if the curved edge is not perfect—you will soon cover this border with another color. Allow to dry, then repeat with a second coat of turquoise polish.

Step 4

When nails are completely dry, use the black striper polish to paint a curved black line between the pink and the yellow layers, as thick or as thin as you want it. Apply to all nails and allow to dry, then apply a second coat if needed.

Step 5

When nails are completely dry, use the red striper polish to paint a curved red line between the pink and turquoise layers, as thick or as thin as you want it. Apply to all nails and allow to dry, then repeat with a second coat if needed.

Step 6

When dry, apply clear top coat and allow the completed look to dry.

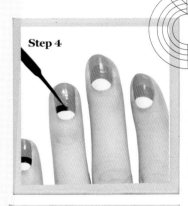

Step 4

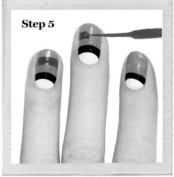

Step 5

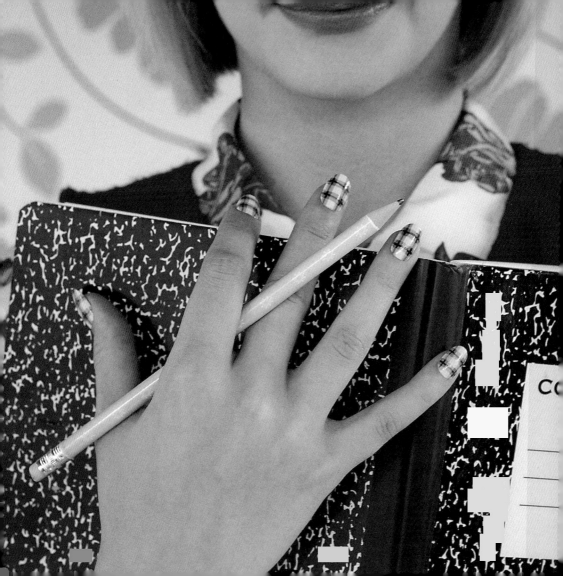

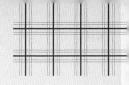

Plaid

Bring out your inner schoolgirl with this traditional motif, perfect for playing hooky or burying yourself in a book. And don't worry about curfew—plaid is playful round-the-clock!

Partner recommended.

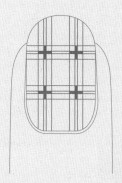

Tools:

☐ Yellow polish

☐ Light gray polish

☐ Dark gray striper polish

☐ Black striper polish

☐ Clear top coat

(continued)

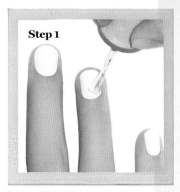

Step 1

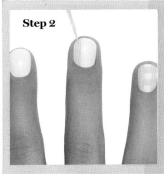

Step 2

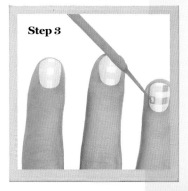

Step 3

Plaid Instructions

Step 1

Apply two coats of yellow polish to all nails and allow to dry after each coat.

Step 2

With the light gray polish, paint two vertical lines and two horizontal lines, creating an evenly spaced grid. Apply to all nails and allow to dry.

Step 3

With the dark gray striper polish, fill in the squares where the vertical and horizontal lines intersect. Apply to all nails and allow to dry.

Step 4

With the dark gray striper polish, paint a thin line down the center of each vertical and horizontal line. Apply to all nails and allow to dry.

Step 5

With the black striper polish, paint a plus sign (+) in the middle of each gray square. Apply to all nails and allow to dry.

Step 6

Apply clear top coat and allow the completed look to dry.

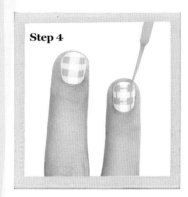

Step 4

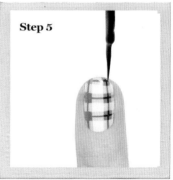

Step 5

Resources

Find more nail art designs on my website (Mpnails.com) and my Twitter and Instagram feeds (both @mpnails). View the work of my amazing friends at Nailing Hollywood (NailingHollywood.com).

Check out my favorite nail polishes—NCLA, Ginger + Liz, RGB, The New Black, Zoya, American Apparel, Orly, and Essie—and get your hands on the number-one top coat, Seche Vite Dry Fast Top Coat, for the fastest drying time and glossiest sheen.

Visit your local retailers—pharmacies, beauty stores, and craft supply outlets—for tools, embellishments, and inspirations, or browse online, starting your search at any one of these online superstores:

For nail care items, polishes, removers, and basic beauty tools, browse **Beauty Bar** (BeautyBar.com) and **Sephora** (Sephora.com).

Online pharmacies like **Walgreens** (Walgreens.com) and **CVS** (CVS.com) have wide selections of nail art products, or try **Sally Beauty** (SallyBeauty.com) and **Nubar** (ByNubar.com) for specific items like stripers, dotting tools, top coats, embellishments, and more.

Jo-Ann Fabric and Craft Stores (JoAnn.com), **Hobby Lobby** (HobbyLobby.com), and **Michaels** (Michaels.com) carry a vast assortment of embellishments and decorative materials.

Acknowledgments

A big thank you to the awesome crew who helped put this book together: to Katie Miller for the instructional photos, to Lara Rossignol for the nail portraits, to the amazing stylists Shiffy Kagan and Ashley Pava, to hair and makeup artists Wendy Osmundson and Hannah Huffy, and to Nasty Gal for the great clothing. Thanks to Maria Minelli's M models: Christina Masterson, Jennifer Christina, and Ika Sharova; and to my hand models and dear friends Kelela Mizanekristos, Amanda Zazi Charchian, Natasha Newman-Thomas, Rico Yves Birden, Natasha Ghosn, Alex Ghosn, and Staz Lindes. Huge thanks to the ladies of Nailing Hollywood—Jenna Hipp, Stephanie Stone, and Vanessa Gualy—and thanks to Jen Gotch, Natalie Shriver, Missy Reno, and Kelly Edmondson for convincing me to become a manicurist. Also, much love to these friends for your support during the making of this book: Tommy Rouse, Vishwam Velandy, Sylvia Kochinski, James Ferraro, Miles Martinez, and Aaron Bondaroff. Finally, thank you to Chronicle Books—to Elizabeth Yarborough and Laura Lee Mattingly—for this opportunity.

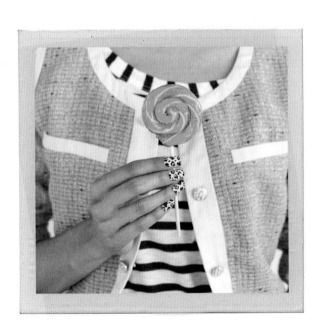